# HYBRID FITNESS ROUTINE

## DISCLAIMER

This book is for general informational purposes only. The author is not a medical professional and nothing in this publication constitutes medical advice. You should consult your physician or other healthcare professional before starting this or any other fitness program to determine if it is right for your needs. This is particularly true if you (or your family) have a history of high blood pressure or heart disease, or if you have ever experienced chest pain when exercising or have experienced chest pain in the past month when not engaged in physical activity. Do not start this fitness program if your physician or healthcare provider advises against it. If you experience faintness, dizziness, pain or shortness of breath at any time while exercising you should stop immediately.

If you choose to use this information without prior consent from your physician, you are agreed to accept full responsibility for your decisions and are agreeing to hold harmless Hybrid Calisthenics, it's agents, contractors, employees, and any affiliated companies from an liability with respect to injury or illness to your or your property arising out of or connected with your use of the information contained within this book.

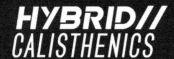

Dedicated to the community and to our wonderful team.

Thank you for making everything possible.

## Acknowledgements

This book was assembled by a team of incredible individuals.

**Maya Brewer -** Fitness Editor
**Gretchen Lents -** Assistant Editor
**Gabriella Nieves -** Book Designer
**Chris  Tully -** Book Designer
**Chrys Johnson -** Fitness Consultant
**Kalyn Cavalier -** Photographer

# TABLE OF CONTENTS

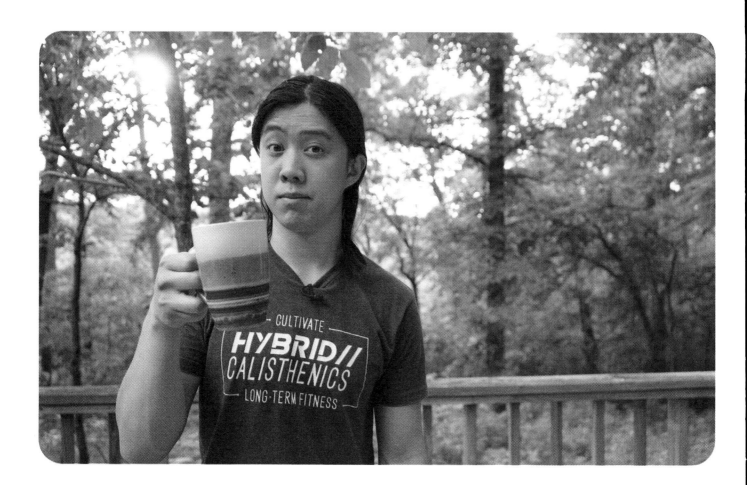

## HELLO FRIEND!

My name is Hampton and I'm the personal trainer that made the fitness routine you'll find in this book. My brand and channel is Hybrid Calisthenics and this fitness routine is commonly referred to as the **Hybrid Routine**.

It's been used by millions of people worldwide, so we'd love to have you on board!

# WHAT'S THE HYBRID ROUTINE?

The Hybrid routine is a fitness routine that uses **progressive bodyweight exercise**. It's designed to help anyone get fit with just their body and gravity! Very little equipment is needed and many exercises don't require any equipment at all.

Every major exercise is also *scalable* – meaning almost anyone can find a variation they can do! Our routine is designed to be for anyone – from young athletes to elderly grandparents.

# WHO IS THIS BOOK FOR?

Well, as mentioned above, the fitness routine can be used by anybody! It's actively being made available in different languages and formats. This is the **book version** of the Hybrid Routine!

For more information, our community and media content can be found as Hybrid Calisthenics on almost every social media platform.

---

Of course, all of this is assuming you don't know me (yet!).

Maybe you got this book as a gift. Or maybe you picked it up as its owner went to the bathroom (in which case, read quickly). I appreciate you all the same.

If you *do* know me and bought this book, then thank you so much! A lot of work went into writing and designing this. I really, really hope you like it.

Let's go!

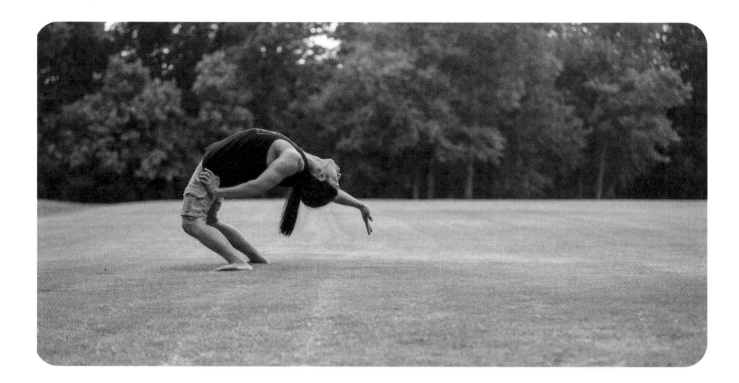

The Hybrid Routine focuses on 6 fundamental movements and makes them progressive. This means their difficulty can be adjusted based on your current fitness level.

So we start with something we can do, and we work our way up as we get stronger!

## Step 1: Fundamental Movements

We're focusing on 6 different exercises that, together, train our entire body. These are:

1. Pushups
2. Pullups
3. Squats
4. Leg Raises
5. Bridges
6. Twists

These mimic the common things we do in life: pushing, pulling, standing up, and more!
While there are other great movements such as lunging and locomotion, the 6 above will give users a wide variety of skills from which they can expand. They're also easily scalable, which plays an important role in home workouts!

## Step 2: Making a Routine

Now that we know our movements, we can schedule these movements into a weekly routine.

A routine is almost always better than doing the exercises "whenever we feel like it." As many trainers say: Consistency is key!

The Hybrid Routine's schedule trains each movement hard twice a week. This gives us a time-efficient routine that allows us to consistently make progress for years. This builds strength and muscle while giving adequate time for rest. Even if you choose to change the routine, I recommend beginners stick with this foundation for at least a few months before moving on.

## Step 3: Progression

Reading Step 1, you might have said "Wait Hampton! I can't do half of these exercises! I'm not strong enough!"

**Great news -** the majority of this book is dedicated to solving this exact problem!
Remember that a key part of the Hybrid Routine is finding a variation suitable for you. So if you can't do Full Pushups yet, try Incline Pushups! If you struggle with Full Pullups, try Horizontal Pullups!

**Using the previous few steps:**
1. You find a variation that you can do safely and pain-free.
2. You work these variations for 2-3 Sets of as many Reps as you can twice a week.
3. When you're able to do a Standard of Sets and Reps, you move on to a harder variation!

Easy peasy, right? The world is your oyster! Unless you don't like oysters, of course.

# WARMING UP

Warming up properly helps us avoid injury and increase performance! A good warmup can enhance our workout. Different warmups work for different people. Some spend a long time warming up and others barely warm up at all! Your need to warm up is affected by factors such as age, physical condition, previous injuries, the current temperature, and more. The warmup below is my suggestion. Over time, experiment with what works best for you!

I prefer a simple two-part warmup:

## Part 1- General Warmup
The purpose here is to just get our blood pumping and muscles moving. We're signaling to our bodies that physical activity is coming! We want our muscles to literally be warm here.

Many different exercises can accomplish this goal:
- Jumping jacks
- Running in place
- Jumping rope
- Arm circles
- Shadowboxing
- ...and more!

Find what works best for you. Start with something gentle if you're uncertain.  Try to warm up your entire body. For example, don't only warm up your arms but neglect your legs!
**Approximate time:** 1-2 Minutes (varies)

## Part 2- Specific Warmup
After our body is nice and warm, it may help to practice an easier variation of the movement(s) you'll do during your main workout.

**For example:**
- if you're about to do Full Pushups, try warming up with Wall Pushups or Incline Pushups!
- If you're about to do Full Squats, try warming up with Assisted Squats or Half Squats!'

If you can't find an easier variation, simply do your workout but with fewer reps. For example, if you're about to do Wall Pushups, you can warm up with Wall Pushups - just do a warmup set of about 50% as many reps as you normally could.
**Approximate time:** 2-5 minutes (varies)

Again, experimentation is key! Don't stress over the "perfect" warmup - it completely depends on the person. If your workouts seem stiff or uncomfortable, you may want to consider a longer warmup.

**We know some people may not be familiar with some of the terms in this book. That's okay! We all start somewhere. Here are some definitions. If you're confused about any term not covered, please email us.**

**Rep:** Short for repetition. The amount of an exercise you do at once. If you do 12 pushups and stop, you did 12 pushup repetitions. Sometimes counted in seconds.

**Set:** A group of reps. If you do 12 pushups, rest, and do 12 more, you did 2 sets of 12 pushups.

**Progression:** A harder version of an exercise, but also used synonymously with "variation" sometimes.

**Regression:** An easier version of an exercise.

**Hampton:** The author of this book and the founder of Hybrid Calisthenics. He loves you.

**Hybrid Calisthenics:** Hampton's brand.

**Calisthenics:** Bodyweight exercise you do with your body and very little equipment.

**Isometrics:** Exercises with no movement. Examples are planks and wall sits.

**Rest Time:** The amount of time between sets.

**Compound Exercise:** An exercise that works multiple muscle groups at once.

**To Failure:** Doing an exercise set until you're unable to do anymore reps.

**Hypertrophy:** Muscle growth.

# HYBRID FITNESS ROUTINE

| Monday | Pushup Progression: 2-3 Sets | Leg Raise Progression: 2-3 Sets |
|---|---|---|
| Tuesday | Pullup Progression: 2-3 Sets | Squat Progression: 2-3 Sets |
| Wednesday | Bridge Progression: 2-3 Sets | Twist Progression: 2-3 Sets |
| Thursday | Pushup Progression: 2-3 Sets | Leg Raise Progression: 2-3 Sets |
| Friday | Pullup Progression: 2-3 Sets | Squat Progression: 2-3 Sets |
| Saturday | Bridge Progression: 2-3 Sets | Twist Progression: 2-3 Sets |
| Sunday | Rest | |

## SIMPLE, EFFICIENT, AND HIGHLY EFFECTIVE

### How to Use

**How Many Reps?** As many as you safely can.

**Repetition Speed:** 2 Seconds Down, 1 Second Pause, 2 Seconds Up, 1 Second Pause.

**Rest Times:** 2-3 Minutes between sets. 5 Minutes between separate exercises.

This program works the entire body and is designed to cover all the most common goals in fitness - strength, muscle, endurance, mobility, toning, and more. It can also help with weight loss OR weight gain depending on how you eat!

When in doubt, start here!

### Sample Workout

For example, after finishing the first set of Pushup Progressions, a user will wait 2-3 minutes before starting their next set. After they finish 2-3 sets of Pushup Progressions, they'll wait 5 minutes before starting on Leg Raises.

Adjust these numbers as needed. They're designed to allow for adequate recovery while still challenging the user. However, they're not set in stone. Feel free to change them up once you're accustomed to the routine!

## What Does "Progression" Mean?

Remember that a key component of this entire book is adjusting each exercise to your current fitness level.

So pick an exercise variation you can do and start with that. When in doubt, **start with the first one.**

For example, **Pushup Progression** could refer to anything from **Wall Pushups** to **Advanced One-Arm Pushups**. I advise everyone to start with Wall Pushups even if they're strong enough to do harder variations. I find it builds better form and healthy movement patterns!

## When to Move on to a Harder Exercise?

You stay on a progression until you're able to reach the Goal Standard of sets and reps.

On each set, we do **as many reps as we safely can.** This is commonly 1–2 reps before failure.

If you consistently do your workouts, your maximum reps will increase over time. Keep in mind that they may not increase every workout and they may not always be even. This is normal!

Once your maximum meets or exceeds the Level 3 Goal Standard for an exercise, you can move on to the next progression!

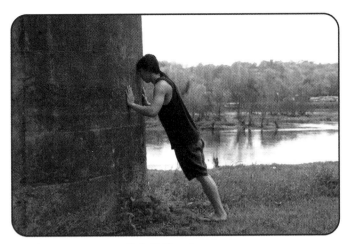

**Wall Pushups**

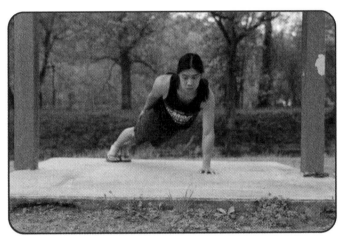

**Advanced One-Arm Pushups**

# HYBRIDIZATION

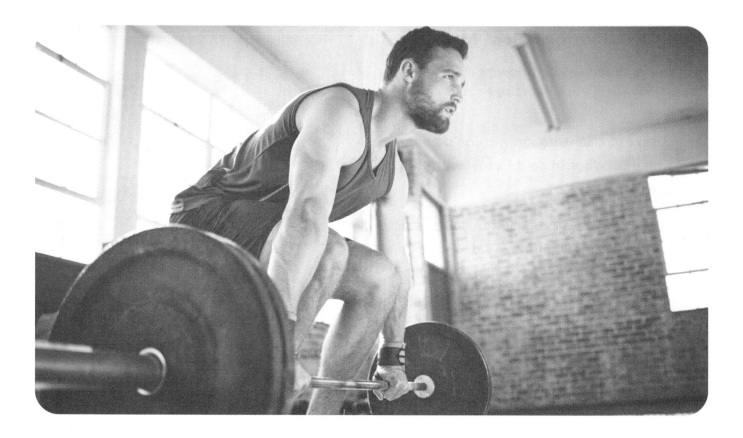

## COMBINING WITH OTHER DISCIPLINES

### "Hampton, can I combine the Hybrid Routine with..."

I get this question all the time. People are interested in combining this routine with anything from barbells to knitting.

The answer is almost always **YES, OF COURSE**!
The Hybrid Routine is designed to build strength, muscle, mobility, and more while leaving room for experimentation.

A common issue I see with fitness routines is that the author assumes – understandably – that the users will follow the routine to the letter. I find this to be very rare! In fact, it's often a struggle getting people to even read all the instructions.

People naturally want to add their own spin to a routine. This makes perfect sense because people have different goals. Some might add jogging whereas others want to add rock climbing. The Hybrid Routine builds a foundation upon which other skills can thrive. That said, some people want to be given exact instructions and/or prefer an efficient workout. You don't have to add anything to the Hybrid Routine. You can follow it to the letter and continue to make progress for years to come. It's up to you!

Here are some things you can combine with the routine:

- Weight Lifting
- Walking, Jogging, or Sprinting
- Yoga
- Tai Chi
- Martial Arts

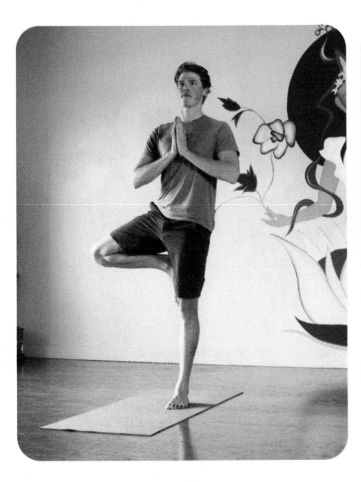 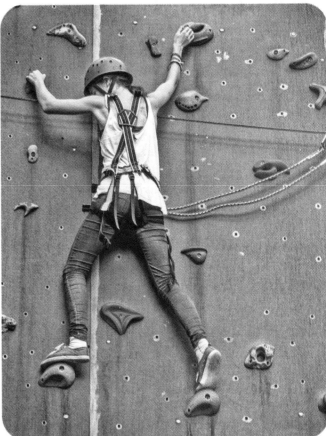

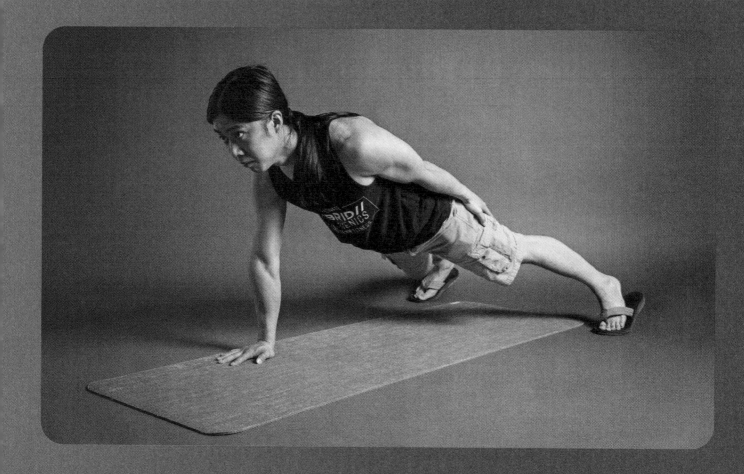

# PUSHUPS

The Pushup is one of the first movements that come to mind when we think about exercise. In fact, pushing is one of our most fundamental movement patterns! Think of pushing a shopping cart, getting up from the floor, raising the roof, and so on. The push pattern is a big part of our daily lives.

That doesn't mean that Pushups are easy. Depending on where you're starting from, the classic Full Pushup can feel quite challenging. That's why we put together this selection of progressions. Start where you are and build up your strength with a healthy movement pattern.

Every variation on a Pushup is a compound movement that works a large muscle group. This exercise utilizes our pectorals, anterior deltoids, and triceps. A number of stabilizing muscles are working throughout the entire movement.

# GENERAL PUSHUP CUES

You may see these cues repeated throughout the exercise variations. This is because they're important, so don't disregard them!

Slow and steady wins the race on this exercise. Don't just speed through these. Find a controlled, rhythmic pace to really feel this movement. 2 Seconds Down, 1 Second Pause, 2 Seconds Up. Repeat.

A good "rule of thumb" is being able to maintain flat palms and feel a slight stretch in your wrist while your arms are straight.

Some people have wrist pain during these exercises. Doing some warmups with the easier variations can help. Stretch your wrists beforehand. If you have a wrist injury, doing these on your knuckles is a temporary solution.

Your core strength will be tested during these exercises. Keep your body firm. Don't let your body arch or sag. Imagine a straight line from the top of your head to your heels. Core strength is important for all calisthenics, and this is great practice!

Film yourself and watch back between sets to check your form. A mirror is also useful.

# PUSHUP PROGRESSIONS

First, we begin pushing against a wall. This simple angle change makes Wall Pushups much easier than Full Pushups. Because of this, we can focus on honing our form and learning a healthy pushing movement.

The angle is slowly increased until we finally touch ground in Knee Pushups! After spending time on this and Full Pushups, we finally start building towards the One-Arm Pushup and beyond! While many claim to be able to do this exercise, many progressions are given here so that readers can build up gradually. This strengthens our joints and builds greater mastery of the movement.

Let's push the limits!

1. Wall Pushups
2. Incline Pushups
3. Advanced Incline Pushups
4. Knee Pushups
5. Full Pushups
6. Narrow Pushups
7. Side-Staggered Pushups
8. Archer Pushups
9. Sliding One-Arm Pushups
10. One-Arm Pushups
11. Advanced One-Arm Pushups

# WALL PUSHUPS

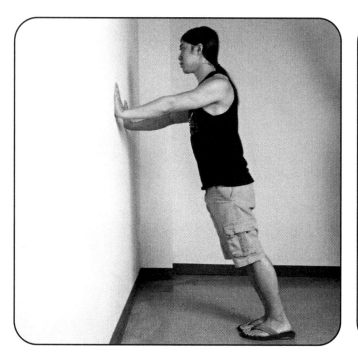

**ASCEND**

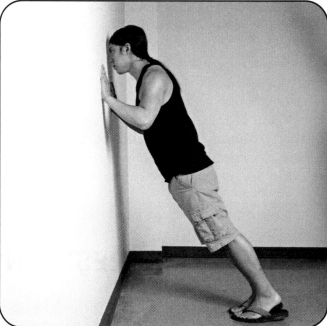

**DESCEND**

## TUTORIAL

1. Stand at arm's length facing a wall.

2. Place your flat palms on the wall. Your arms should be straight.

3. Descend slowly until your head gently touches the wall.

4. Pause for 1 second.

5. Slowly come back up.

6. Pause for 1 second.

7. Repeat.

## STANDARDS

**LEVEL 1:** 2 sets of 30
**LEVEL 2:** 2 sets of 50
**LEVEL 3:** 3 sets of 50

Do 2-3 sets of as many as you can.

Once you can meet or exceed Level 3 with **GOOD FORM,** you are ready to move on to a harder variation.

# BEHIND THE EXERCISE

One of the easiest pushing movements, this exercise is an incredible start to our Pushup series. The high angle makes this movement a lot easier than Full Pushups.

Although often considered "too easy" by seasoned athletes and total beginners alike, almost anyone can benefit from a few sets of Wall Pushups. The low resistance allows the user to really focus on form - which builds healthy movement patterns for our harder variations!

They're also a great therapy exercise. The gentle movement stretches stiff muscles and heals old wounds.

When in doubt, start here!

# FORM CUES

Slow and steady wins the race on this exercise. Don't just speed through these. Find a controlled, rhythmic, pace to really feel this movement. 2 seconds down, 1 second pause, 2 seconds up. Repeat.

Keep your hands around chest height. Hands placed too high put more work on our elbows than we need at the moment. Hands placed too low make it difficult to keep our palms flat. A good "rule of thumb" is being able to maintain flat palms and feel a slight stretch in your wrist while your arms are straight.

Keep your body firm. Don't arch your body at the bottom to make the motion easier. Core strength is important for all calisthenics, and this is a great place to start building it.

# PROGRESSION & REGRESSION

**To make this exercise harder:** Do these through a doorframe or gymnastic rings to increase range of motion. Descend until you are unable to descend further before coming back up.

**To make this exercise easier:** Doing these on your knees will make them easier. However, because wall pushups are only slightly harder than opening doors, you may have better results with doing fewer wall pushups at first, rather than making them easier.

# INCLINE PUSHUPS

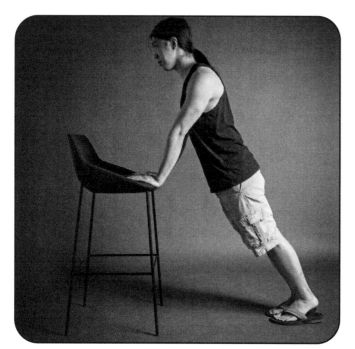

**ASCEND**

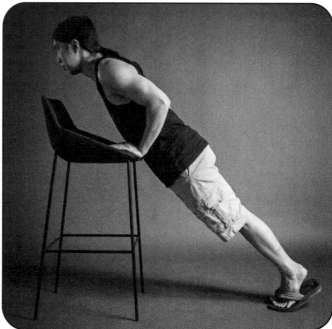

**DESCEND**

## TUTORIAL

1. Stand facing your base – it should be approximately sternum height.

2. Lean forward and place your hands on the base. Your arms should be straight.

3. Descend slowly until your chest gently touches the base. Your hands may brush your chest.

4. Pause for 1 second.

5. Slowly come back up.

6. Pause for 1 second.

7. Repeat.

## STANDARDS

**LEVEL 1:** 2 sets of 20
**LEVEL 2:** 2 sets of 30
**LEVEL 3:** 3 sets of 40

Do 2-3 sets of as many as you can.

Once you can meet or exceed Level 3 with **GOOD FORM,** you are ready to move on to a harder variation.

# BEHIND THE EXERCISE

After we've mastered Wall Pushups, it's time to start increasing resistance! We can do this by decreasing the angle of our starting position.

Incline Pushups get us closer to the ground and introduce us to diagonal pushing. You will feel the difference in the workload as you change your angle, and you may begin to notice the increased demand on your core for stability. The lower the surface you are pushing off of, the harder the exercise will be!

Start off with something around sternum height. Some commonly used surfaces include counter tops, support railings, and even the trunk of a mid-sized sedan. Just make sure the car is parked first!

# FORM CUES

You may not be able to find something exactly at sternum height. That's okay. Work with what you have. Just make sure the base is safe and secure. Safety first! You can push the object against a wall for extra stability.

Like with Wall Pushups, how you position your hands relative to your body makes a difference. At the bottom position of the exercise, your hands should be next to your chest. If they're by your shoulders, try to move your feet closer or find a slightly lower base.

Your core strength begins to get tested here. Keep your body firm and straight. Don't let your lower back sag. These earlier variations will help build a solid foundation for the harder Pushups!

Keep your arms approximately shoulder width apart.

Keep your feet together.

# PROGRESSION & REGRESSION

**To make this exercise harder:** A lower base makes this exercise harder.

**To make this exercise easier:** A higher base makes this exercise easier.

# ADVANCED INCLINE PUSHUPS

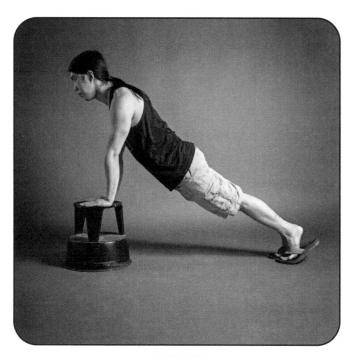

**ASCEND**

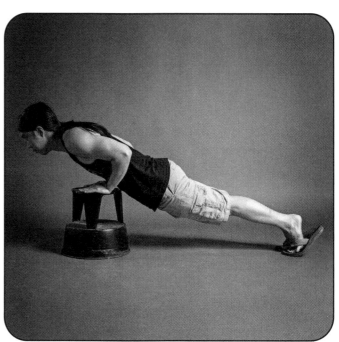

**DESCEND**

## TUTORIAL

1. Stand facing your base – it should be approximately hip height.

2. Lean forward and place your hands on the base. Your arms should be straight.

3. Descend slowly until your chest gently touches the base. Your hands may brush your chest.

4. Pause for 1 second.

5. Slowly come back up.

6. Pause for 1 second.

7. Repeat.

## STANDARDS

**LEVEL 1:** 2 sets of 20
**LEVEL 2:** 2 sets of 30
**LEVEL 3:** 3 sets of 35

Do 2-3 sets of as many as you can.

Once you can meet or exceed Level 3 with **GOOD FORM,** you are ready to move on to a harder variation.

# BEHIND THE EXERCISE

This is a natural step after regular Incline Pushups. Lowering the base makes this exercise noticeably harder.

This is when your core strength becomes much more important. You will need this core strength to do regular Full Pushups. If you reach Full Pushups and realize you cannot do it with an aligned body, revisit this exercise. Use a lower base if necessary. Build alignment with this step.

The standard for this step is a base around hip height. Feel free to adjust the height of the base as necessary. Some commonly used surfaces include the arm of a couch, the seat of a sturdy chair, and a park bench. If you have gymnastic rings, you can lower the straps an inch or two every week as you get stronger - provided you can maintain solid form!

# FORM CUES

Filming yourself and watching back is a good idea for all exercises, but especially this one. You can even review your form as you're resting between sets. If your butt is too high or your lower back is sagging, adjust as needed and try again!

You may not be able to find something exactly at hip height. That's okay. Work with what you have. Just make sure the base is safe and secure. Safety first! You can push the object against a wall for extra stability.

Like with Wall Pushups, how you position your hands relative to your body makes a difference. At the bottom position of the exercise, your hands should be next to your chest. If they're by your shoulders, try to move your feet closer or find a slightly lower base.

Your core strength begins to get tested here. Keep your body firm and straight. Don't let your lower back sag. These earlier variations will help build a solid foundation for the harder Pushups!

Keep your arms approximately shoulder width apart.

Keep your feet together.

# PROGRESSION & REGRESSION

**To make this exercise harder:** A lower base makes this exercise harder. Or you can bring your hands closer together.

**To make this exercise easier:** A higher base makes this exercise easier. Or you can do these on your knees, if you have an object around knee height.

# KNEE PUSHUPS

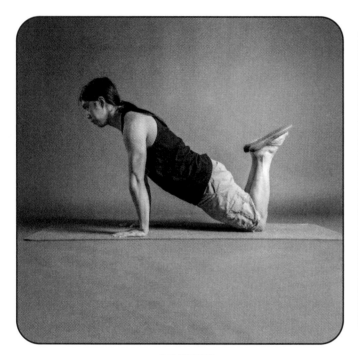

**ASCEND**

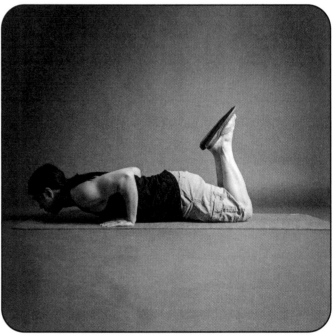

**DESCEND**

## TUTORIAL

1. Kneel on the floor with your knees together.

2. Lean forward and place your hands on the ground. Your arms should be straight and your body aligned from your head to knees.

3. Descend slowly until your chest gently touches the floor. Your hands may brush your chest.

4. Pause for 1 second.

5. Slowly come back up.

6. Pause for 1 second.

7. Repeat.

## STANDARDS

**LEVEL 1:** 2 sets of 10
**LEVEL 2:** 2 sets of 20
**LEVEL 3:** 3 sets of 30

Do 2-3 sets of as many as you can.

Once you can meet or exceed Level 3 with **GOOD FORM,** you are ready to move on to a harder variation.

## BEHIND THE EXERCISE

With this step, we're finally touching ground for Horizontal Pushups! We're almost to the iconic Full Pushup. The modification is simple - because we're pushing from our knees instead of our toes as a pivot, less weight is being moved.

While the pushing demands are greater, some might find the core demands of this exercise easier than the previous step (Advanced Incline Pushups). Feel free to add a few aligned exercises at the end of your workout to maintain your core strength.

Some guys are hesitant to do this exercise because they're called "girl pushups" in some school gym classes. Ignore this. There are many Pushup variations. Some are much easier than Knee Pushups. Some are much harder than Full Pushups.

Temporarily remove ego from your training and build up with this excellent exercise for both strength and therapy.

## FORM CUES

For some reason, it's common to let the lower back sag during this exercise. Do your best to keep your body aligned from your head to your knees.

Place your hands below your chest. They shouldn't be too far towards your head or towards your knees. Find the balance.

Some people have wrist pain during this exercise. Doing some warmups with the easier variations can help. Stretch your wrists beforehand.

Keep your arms approximately shoulder width apart.

Keep your knees together.

# PROGRESSION & REGRESSION

**To make this exercise harder:** Lowering down on your knees and coming up on your toes makes this exercise harder.

**To make this exercise easier:** A higher base makes this exercise easier. Even a few blocks can help.

# FULL PUSHUPS

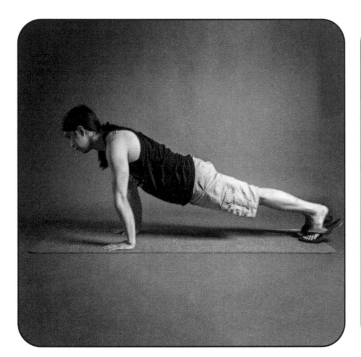

**ASCEND**

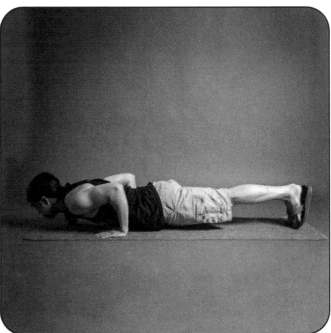

**DESCEND**

## TUTORIAL

1. Kneel on the floor with your knees together.

2. Lean forward and place your hands on the ground. Straighten your knees. Your arms should be straight and your body aligned from your head to your knees.

3. Descend slowly until your chest gently touches the floor. Your hands may brush your chest.

4. Pause for 1 second.

5. Slowly come back up.

6. Pause for 1 second.

7. Repeat.

## STANDARDS

**LEVEL 1:** 2 sets of 5
**LEVEL 2:** 2 sets of 15
**LEVEL 3:** 3 sets of 25

Do 2-3 sets of as many as you can.

Once you can meet or exceed Level 3 with **GOOD FORM,** you are ready to move on to a harder variation.

# BEHIND THE EXERCISE

Here it is! This is the famous Full Pushup - used across the world by anyone from athletes to astronauts. It's quite possibly the most famous calisthenics exercise ever.

That said, while many CLAIM to be able to do these with ease, it's relatively uncommon to see the average person do several Full Pushups with good form.

This exercise utilizes the largest muscle group in the upper body, and the increased strength demand will become apparent immediately! Master this exercise with an aligned body and proper range of motion.

Your upper body strength, core strength, and joint health will be all the better for it! You'll also put on some muscle as well.

# FORM CUES

You might be tempted to sag your lower body or chest. This makes this exercise easier by allowing you to touch your chest despite not descending as deeply. Keep your body aligned from your head to your feet!

Film yourself and watch back between sets to check your form. A mirror is also useful.

Place your hands below your chest. They shouldn't be too far towards your head or towards your knees. Find the balance.

Some people have wrist pain during this exercise. Doing some warmups with the easier variations can help. Stretch your wrists beforehand.

If you have a wrist injury, doing these on your knuckles is a temporary solution.

Keep your arms approximately shoulder width apart.

Keep your feet together.

# PROGRESSION & REGRESSION

**To make this exercise harder:** Doing this exercise slower can make it significantly harder for some trainees - especially the ones used to relying on momentum. Better strength and muscle can be built by controlling every inch of the movement.

**To make this exercise easier:** Doing this exercise at a slight incline can make it easier. This is basically going back to Incline Pushups, but with a base only a foot or two off the ground (30-60 cm). A stool or ottoman pushed against a wall works well.

# NARROW PUSHUPS

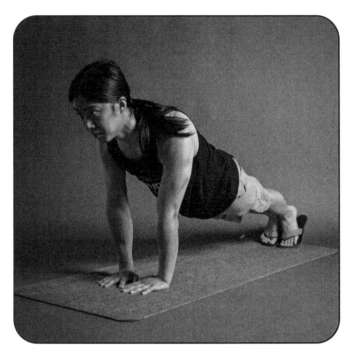

**ASCEND**

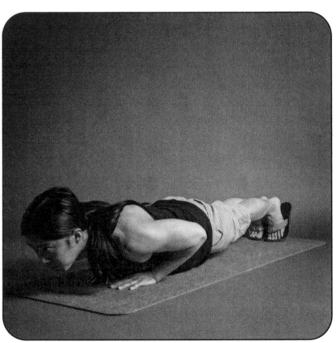

**DESCEND**

## TUTORIAL

1. Kneel on the floor with your knees together.

2. Lean forward and place your hands on the ground. The tip of your index fingers should be touching.

3. Straighten your knees. Your arms should be straight and your body aligned from your head to your knees.

4. Descend slowly until your chest gently touches the floor. Your hands may brush your chest.

5. Pause for 1 second.

6. Slowly come back up.

7. Pause for 1 second.

8. Repeat 4–7.

## STANDARDS

**LEVEL 1:** 2 sets of 5
**LEVEL 2:** 2 sets of 10
**LEVEL 3:** 3 sets of 20

Do 2-3 sets of as many as you can.

Once you can meet or exceed Level 3 with **GOOD FORM,** you are ready to move on to a harder variation.

# BEHIND THE EXERCISE

Now that we have worked Full Pushups thoroughly, we can start training our body for harder pushing exercises.

(You HAVE worked Full Pushups and are able to at least do Level 3 of them, right? If not, go back and work them! You'll make better progress that way).

Moving our hands closer together gives more work to our arms. Although the pectorals are often emphasized in modern training, the "weak link" of our pushing movements is usually our arms. This is why our routine is dedicated to building them up - a chain is only as strong as its weakest link!

Very importantly, this step begins conditioning our elbows and shoulders for the rigors of one-arm work.

Fear not though, all the remaining exercises still heavily work our chest muscles. In fact, with Narrow Pushups, our pectorals are actually much closer to peak contraction than in Full Pushups!

# FORM CUES

Your thumbs don't have to form a "diamond." Doing this flares your elbows a bit more, which increases pectoral activation. However, if this irritates your elbow, you can tuck your thumbs in for now. Just touch your index fingers together. You can always come back to this when you're stronger.

If touching the tip of your index fingers is too difficult, simply start with a Full Pushup and move your hands a few inches closer together. Work these until you feel strong enough to move them closer again. Repeat.

Keep your body aligned. Don't sag!

Film yourself and watch back between sets to check your form. A mirror is also useful.

Place your hands below your chest. They shouldn't be too far towards your head or towards your knees. Find the balance.

Some people have wrist pain during this exercise. Doing some warmups with the easier variations can help. Stretch your wrists beforehand.

Keep your feet together.

# PROGRESSION & REGRESSION

**To make this exercise harder:** Moving your hands closer together - even to the point where one hand is on TOP of the other - can make this exercise more difficult.

**To make this exercise easier:** Keeping your hands further apart make this exercise easier. Moving them a few inches closer to each other every few weeks can be a steady way to build up to Narrow Pushups.

# SIDE STAGGERED PUSHUPS

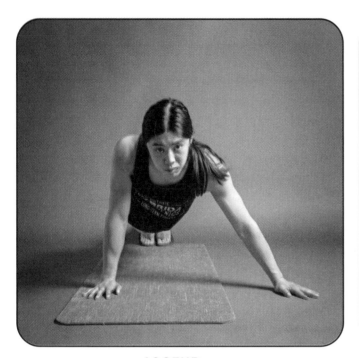

**ASCEND**

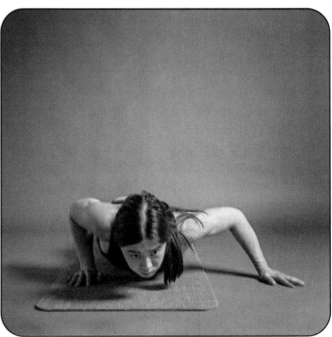

**DESCEND**

## TUTORIAL

1. Kneel on the floor with your knees together.

2. Lean forward and place your hands on the ground. Place your working hand under your chest and your assisting arm 2 palms' length away from your torso.

3. Straighten your knees. Your arms should be straight and your body aligned from your head to your knees.

4. Descend straight down slowly until your chest gently touches the floor. Your working hand may brush your chest.

5. Pause for 1 second.

6. Slowly come back up.

7. Pause for 1 second.

8. Repeat 4-7.

## STANDARDS

**LEVEL 1:** 2 sets of 5 (per side)
**LEVEL 2:** 2 sets of 10 (per side)
**LEVEL 3:** 2 sets of 20 (per side)

Do 2-3 sets of as many as you can.

Once you can meet or exceed Level 3 with **GOOD FORM,** you are ready to move on to a harder variation.

# BEHIND THE EXERCISE

After becoming well-versed with bilateral pushing, we can now officially begin assisted one-arm work. But we're not going to just dive straight into One Arm Pushups! We still have some progressions to move through first.

It's like learning to ride a bike. Most of us had to use training wheels for a while before we graduated to a grown-up bike! In a similar sense, we are preparing our bodies for more complex work by slowly challenging our single-arm strength and stability.

Having one arm further away gives more work to our working arm. Push with as much emphasis on your working arm as you can while letting your "kickstand" arm support and stabilize the movement.

# FORM CUES

Try to go straight up and down. If you find yourself leaning towards your assisting arm, then simply bring it closer until you're able to go straight up and down. Leaning makes the exercise easier.

Start with your assisting arm 2 palms' length away from your torso. Adjust as needed.

Keep your body aligned. Don't sag!

Film yourself and watch back between sets to check your form. A mirror is also useful.

Keep your feet together.

# PROGRESSION & REGRESSION

**To make this exercise harder:** Moving your supporting arm further away makes this exercise harder. Doing this exercise with a straight assisting arm can be quite difficult. Be sure to go straight up and down. Moving side-to-side would turn this into a variation of Archer Pushups - which is explored later in our Pushup series.

**To make this exercise easier:** Moving your assisting hand closer to your torso will make this exercise easier. Don't move it too close, or you'll just be doing Full Pushups. If you're unable to maintain good form with your assisting hand 1 palm length away from your torso, spend some more time on Narrow Pushups.

# ARCHER PUSHUPS

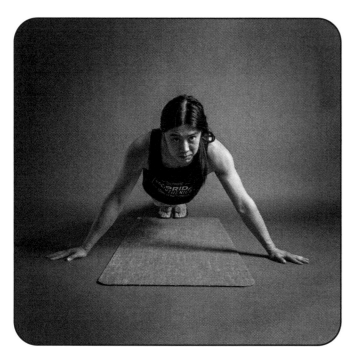

**ASCEND**

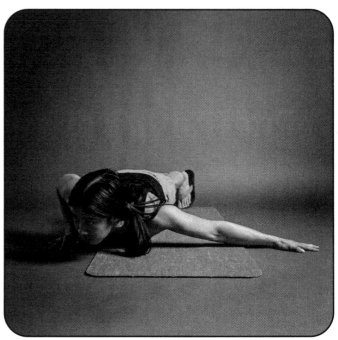

**DESCEND**

## TUTORIAL

1. Kneel on the floor with your knees together.

2. Lean forward and place your hands twice shoulder length width on the ground.

3. Straighten your knees. Your arms should be straight and your body aligned from your head to knees.

4. Keeping your support arm straight, descend towards your working hand slowly until your chest gently touches the floor. Your working hand may brush your chest.

5. Pause for 1 second.

6. Slowly come back up.

7. Pause for 1 second.

8. Repeat 4-7.

# STANDARDS

**LEVEL 1:** 2 sets of 5 (per side)
**LEVEL 2:** 2 sets of 9 (per side)
**LEVEL 3:** 2 sets of 12 (per side)

Do 2-3 sets of as many as you can.

Once you can meet or exceed Level 3 with **GOOD FORM,** you are ready to move on to a harder variation.

# BEHIND THE EXERCISE

The previous step started teaching our nervous system the feeling of one-sided pushing. This next step increases the resistance by leaning more to one side!

Increasing the distance between your hands increases the strength demands on the working arm to a higher degree. This more dramatic lean into the working arm teaches the body to rely less and less on the kickstand arm.

Some people feel increased pressure on their wrists as they work through unilateral pushups. Try to distribute the weight evenly throughout your hand and fingertip on both sides.

# FORM CUES

Work one side at a time to maintain time under tension.

Unlike the Side-Staggered Pushups, we DON'T want to go straight up and down. Lean heavily towards your working arm.

Start with your arms twice shoulder width. Ideally, both arms would be straight at the beginning.

Do your best to keep your body aligned from your feet to your head. Your hips may lean one way at first. Straighten over time.

Film yourself and watch back between sets to check your form. A mirror is also useful.

Keep your feet together.

# PROGRESSION & REGRESSION

**To make this exercise harder:** Perfecting your form in this exercise makes it particularly difficult. Maintain a straight, aligned body while keeping your supporting arm straight. Film yourself and watch back to keep yourself honest. If this becomes too easy, start exploring the next step: Sliding One-Arm Pushups.

**To make this exercise easier:** Moving your hands closer together will make this exercise easier. Keeping your supporting arm bent will also help.

# SLIDING ONE ARM PUSHUPS

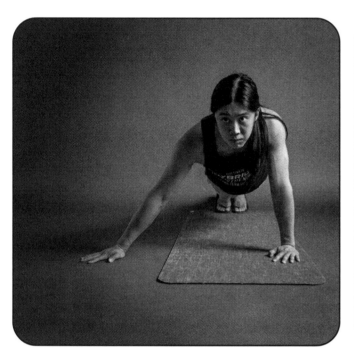

**ASCEND**

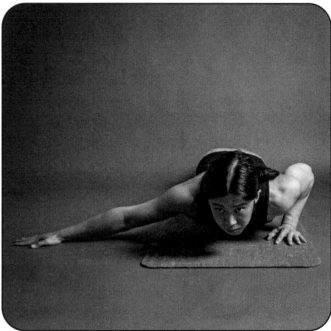

**DESCEND**

## TUTORIAL

1. Kneel on the floor with your knees together.

2. Lean forward and place your hands on the ground. One underneath your chest (like in full pushups) and the other held away from your body.

3. Straighten your knees. Your arms should be straight and your body aligned from your head to your knees.

4. Descend straight down slowly until your chest gently touches the floor. Your working hand may brush your chest.

5. Pause for 1 second.

6. Slowly come back up.

7. Pause for 1 second.

8. Repeat 4-7.

## STANDARDS

**LEVEL 1:** 2 sets of 5 (per side)
**LEVEL 2:** 2 sets of 9 (per side)
**LEVEL 3:** 2 sets of 12 (per side)

Do 2-3 sets of as many as you can.

Once you can meet or exceed Level 3 with **GOOD FORM,** you are ready to move on to a harder variation.

# BEHIND THE EXERCISE

This exercise is similar to Archer Pushups. The difference is that the user goes straight up and down, allowing their supporting arm to slide away at the bottom range. We're one step away from removing the kickstand entirely!

The moving supporting arm challenges our stability. Not only does this increase resistance for the working arm, but it helps build the balance and core strength required for One-Arm Pushups.

This will require more targeted awareness of the movement pattern throughout the exercise. Remember, the motion should be straight up and down. Work hard to minimize any side-to-side shifting.

# FORM CUES

Work one side at a time to maintain time under tension.

Go straight up and down. If your body starts to lean towards your supporting arm, concentrate on tensing your core muscles to bring it back straight.

Start with your arms twice shoulder width apart, then move your working hand under your chest.

Do your best to keep your body aligned from your feet to your head. Your hips may lean one way at first. Straighten over time.

Film yourself and watch back between sets to check your form. A mirror is also useful.

Keep your feet together.

# PROGRESSION & REGRESSION

**To make this exercise harder:** Subtly reducing the assistance from your supporting arm will make this exercise noticeably more difficult. You'll notice that your hip will eventually drift towards your working side. This is unavoidable because of balance issues.

**To make this exercise easier:** Assisting with a bent arm will make this exercise easier.

# ONE ARM PUSHUPS

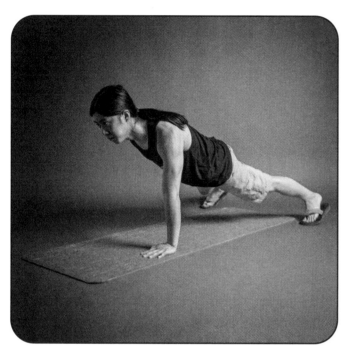

**ASCEND**

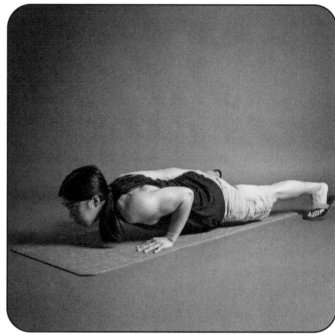

**DESCEND**

## TUTORIAL

1. Kneel on the floor with your knees shoulder width apart.

2. Lean foward and place one hand on the ground. Place the other on your thigh.

3. Straighten your knees. Your working arm should be straight and your body aligned from your head to your hips.

4. Descend straight down slowly until your chest gently touches the floor. Your working hand may brush your chest.

5. Pause for 1 second.

6. Slowly come back up.

7. Pause for 1 second.

8. Repeat 4-7.

# STANDARDS

**LEVEL 1:** 2 sets of 3 (per side)
**LEVEL 2:** 2 sets of 6 (per side)
**LEVEL 3:** 2 sets of 9 (per side)

Do 2-3 sets of as many as you can.

Once you can meet or exceed Level 3 with **GOOD FORM,** you are ready to move on to a harder variation.

# BEHIND THE EXERCISE

This is the legendary exercise used to demonstrate and build strength! Because of its simplicity, its origins probably go back many millennia.

While many CLAIM to be able to do this exercise with ease, very few can do it with good form.

Mastering every inch of this movement will give you exceptional core and unilateral pushing strength.

Done for medium to high reps, this will also build significant muscle to dedicated users.

Congratulations on making it to this step!

# FORM CUES

Keep your feet a bit wider than shoulder width. This is the first Pushup variation in this series where your feet aren't together. This is for balance reasons.

Work one side at a time to maintain time under tension.

Try to keep your shoulders parallel to the ground. Tilting your non-working shoulder away from the ground can make this movement much easier. This is okay at first. Over time, level out your shoulders.

Try to go straight up and down. Even very strong athletes sometimes have a slight shift at the bottom. This is weakness in this range of motion. Again, it may be unavoidable at first. Control it over time.

# PROGRESSION & REGRESSION

**To make this exercise harder:** Moving your feet closer together will make this exercise more difficult.

**To make this exercise easier:** As mentioned above, tilting your non-working shoulder away makes this exercise easier. Use this to built up some reps if necessary, but straighten out your shoulders over time. Alternatively, you can also do these on a short ledge, essentially doing Incline One-Arm Pushups!

# ADVANCED ONE ARM PUSHUPS

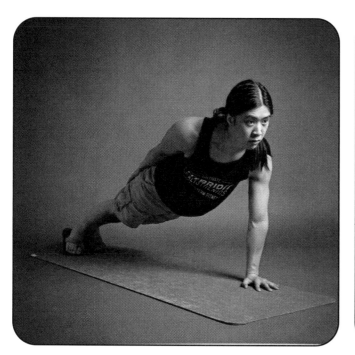

**ASCEND**

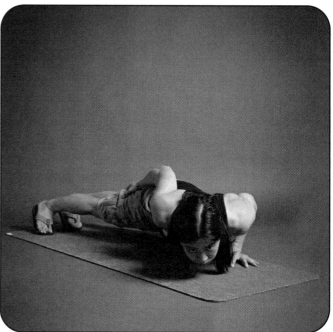

**DESCEND**

## TUTORIAL

1. Kneel on the floor with your knees together.

2. Lean forward and place one hand on the ground. Place the other on your thigh.

3. Straighten your knees. Your working arm should be straight and your body aligned from your head to your feet. Your heels should touch.

4. Descend straight down slowly until your chest gently touches the floor. Your working hand may brush your chest. Your body will be curved.

5. Pause for 1 Second.

6. Slowly come back up.

7. Pause for 1 Second.

8. Repeat 4-7.

# STANDARDS

**LEVEL 1:** 2 sets of 3 (per side)
**LEVEL 2:** 2 sets of 6 (per side)
**LEVEL 3:** 2 sets of 9 (per side)

Do 2-3 sets of as many as you can.

Once you can meet or exceed Level 3 with **GOOD FORM,** you are ready to move on to a harder variation.

# BEHIND THE EXERCISE

This is a rarely seen Pushup variation that can bring excellent results to those who master it.

Bringing our feet together increases the resistance on our working arm. Our waist has to twist a bit towards our working side to balance this.

The sides of our body also get significant work. Expect soreness!

# FORM CUES

Keep your feet together and allow your waist to twist towards your working side. Balance will require you to twist more on the descent.

Try to keep your shoulders parallel to the ground. Tilting your non-working shoulder away from the ground can make this movement much easier. This is okay at first. Over time, level out your shoulders.

Try to go straight up and down. Even very strong athletes sometimes have a slight shift at the bottom. This is weakness in this range of motion. Again, it may be unavoidable at first. Control it over time.

Film yourself and watch back between sets to check your form. A mirror is also useful.

Keep your feet together.

# PROGRESSION & REGRESSION

**To make this exercise harder:** Moving your hand closer to beneath your sternum will exponentially increase this exercise's difficulty. Your body will twist less from this angle. Doing this with a fully aligned body with the hand underneath the sternum is one of the hardest bodyweight pushing exercises in the world. I haven't seen this done on video before.

**To make this exercise easier:** Keeping your feet slightly apart will make this exercise easier.

# CLOSING THOUGHTS

That's the Pushup series for now! If you made it through the entire series, you've built strong, athletic pushing power. Great work!

As you go about your day, take notice of all the ways that a good pushing pattern comes into play. Maybe you're rearranging the furniture in your living room. Perhaps you are pushing a child (or a child at heart!) on a swing set at the local playground. As you notice these pushing movements throughout your day, remember to thank yourself for dedicating time to such a fundamental movement pattern.

So, where do you go from there? Well, you can explore dips, adding weight, or other pushing variations! Here are a few interesting variations you may want to try:

**Dips** – You can do this classic exercise just about anywhere! You can use a couch, a park bench, parallel bars, the bumper of a sedan – you can even do this exercise on the floor! This exercise will supplement your pushups by training your chest, triceps and shoulders. Like pushups, there are many types of dips. Find a variation that works for you!

Be cautious when trying this exercise for the first time, as it can put extra strain on your shoulders. Start by doing dips from the floor (the lowest possible base of support) and slowly working your way to raised surfaces. As it is with every exercise, you should master the simplest variations first before moving on to the next progression.

**Explosive Pushups** – This exercise takes pushups to the next level by adding the element of explosive power. When you lower down, you are building up potential energy, which will allow you to "explode" upward – your hands will leave the ground entirely! Many people aim to add a mid-air clap to this exercise, just for fun. Be careful that you don't land on your face!

**Handstand Pushups** – These are a great shoulder exercise for those that can do them safely! As you can imagine, this exercise requires a lot of practice to develop the right skillset. Balance, core strength, and arm strength will be very important, as will the ability to get in and out of this inverted position safely. An easier variation is Pike Pushups. Both are useful for training vertical pushing!

---

There's a phrase I want you to consider: "Practice does not make perfect. Only perfect practice makes perfect." This doesn't mean we need to overthink. However, don't take shortcuts when learning how to do this exercise. Valuable progressions are often skipped for being "too easy." Skills take consistent practice to develop – make sure your practice is perfect by using a progression you can do well!

**Where do I start?**

Start with a variation that you can do competently with good form for at least a few repetitions. When in doubt, start with Wall Pushups!

**Pushups are hard on my wrists. What should I do?**

You have a few options. The first thing to try is warming up your wrists! Make some gentle wrist circles going one way. After 10 to 20 seconds, switch directions.

If this doesn't help, you might try doing pushups on your fists. There are also devices called pushup handles, or pushup bars, that can take pressure off your wrists during the exercise. You can also hold dumbbells or parallettes.

**I have met the standard for one variation, but the next exercise feels too hard. What should I do?**

Each exercise has a Progression and a Regression. You can use these to your advantage!

For example, let's say you are stuck somewhere between two exercises. If your Wall Pushups are too easy, the Progression will challenge your body in preparation for the next exercise (use a doorframe or gym rings).

Alternatively, if the Incline Pushups are too challenging, the Regression will allow you to build into them more slowly (use a higher base).

You can think of these as transition exercises!

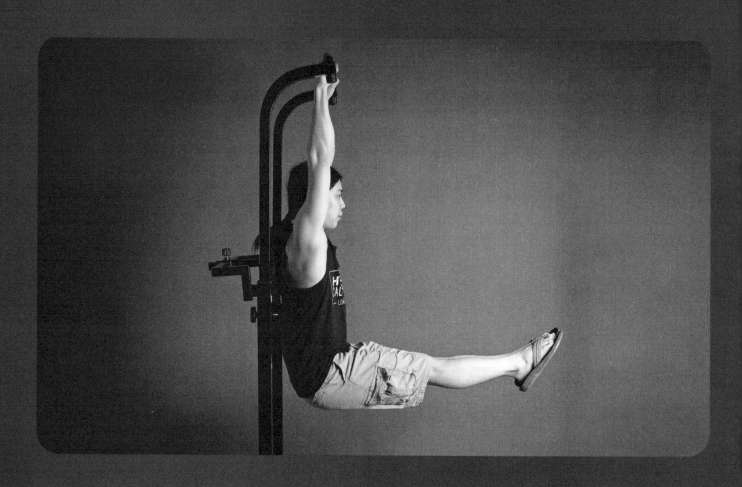

# LEG RAISES

The Leg Raise is a fantastic exercise for strengthening your core. This exercise is extremely scalable. On one end, you might encounter an exercise like a Dead Bug during physical therapy. On the other end, you might find yourself in a Clutch Flag like an absolute champion! Within such a wide range, the possibilities are endless.

Our core strength is leveraged in almost every movement, hold, and function we perform.

Improving core strength with leg raises can help in a wide variety of daily tasks. In addition, we raise our legs when we run, jump, kick, and more! This is a useful pattern to learn.

With proper form, Leg Raises work muscle groups throughout your whole body, including the rectus abdominis, hip flexor muscles, hamstrings, and lower back muscles. A number of stabilizing muscles are working throughout the entire movement.

# GENERAL LEG RAISE CUES

Keep your core engaged with each Leg Raise variation. Imagine bracing yourself for a punch – you should feel the muscles in your core tense up to support you. You could also imagine pulling your bellybutton in and up towards your heart.

Don't forget to breathe! Exhale during the "working" phase of the exercise.

Keeping your thighs pressed together may help you focus on the movement.

The more you extend your knees, the harder these exercises will be!

If your lower back hurts, using a small pillow or small rolled up towel underneath your lower back is a temporary solution.

Film yourself and watch back between sets to check your form. A mirror is also useful!

# LEG RAISE PROGRESSIONS

We'll begin with our bent-knee variations. These early progressions are the safest place to learn to maintain good pelvic positioning. Don't move on to the next progressions until you can meet the standards without pain or discomfort.

Once we have mastered the bent-knee variations, we can move onto Full Leg Raises! This is a calisthenics standard that challenges the abdominals and hip flexors. The following progressions will begin to challenge mobility as well as strength.

Finally, we'll get vertical with it! Beginning with Hanging Knee Raises, you'll build upper body strength while introducing the element of gravity to your core work. Eventually, you'll be able to bring those toes ABOVE your head with the impressive Toe to Bars exercise.

Let's raise the limits!

1. Knee Raises
2. Advanced Knee Raises
3. Alternating Leg Raises
4. Full Leg Raises
5. Tuck Plow Raises
6. Plow Raises
7. Hanging Knee Raises
8. Advanced Hanging Knee Raises
9. Hanging Leg Raises
10. Toe to Bars

# KNEE RAISES

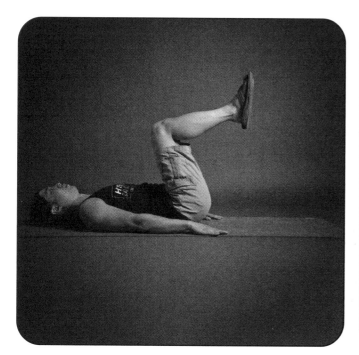

**ASCEND**

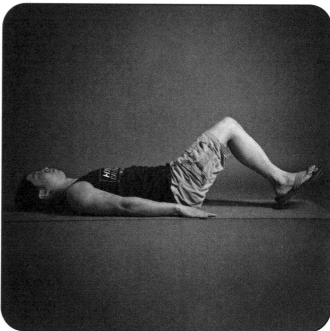

**DESCEND**

## TUTORIAL

1. Lie flat on the floor with your arms by your side.

2. Bend your knees until they are approximately 90 degrees.

3. Bring your legs up until your knees are over your waist. Control the movement.

4. Pause for 1 Second, feeling the contraction in your hips and abs.

5. Slowly descend while straightening your legs until your heels are about 1 inch off the ground.

6. Pause for 1 Second.

7. Repeat 3-6.

# STANDARDS

**LEVEL 1:** 2 sets of 10
**LEVEL 2:** 2 sets of 20
**LEVEL 3:** 2 sets of 30

Do 2-3 sets of as many as you can.

Once you can meet or exceed Level 3 with **GOOD FORM,** you are ready to move on to a harder variation.

# BEHIND THE EXERCISE

Our Leg Raise series focuses on strengthening the waist in conjunction with the hips. This is rooted in the fundamental nature of how we usually use these muscles. Running, jumping, and kicking all involve synergy between our core and hips. It's common to bring our legs up towards our upper body (like in Leg Raises). This is one of the few reasons why Leg Raises are used in our routine over Sit ups.

Knee Raises are a great place to begin our journey!

Bending the knees will make this exercise fundamentally easier than regular Leg Raises. In addition, we are unable to descend as far as we would with straight legs - our feet get in the way!

That said, the bottom part of this exercise is still the most difficult. Try not to let your heels touch the floor. Pause an inch above the ground before reversing the movement. While you may dislike this at first, this will build excellent isometric strength you'll need for the more advanced progressions!

# FORM CUES

Keep your heels off the ground throughout the exercise. Touching the ground at the bottom of the movement makes this exercise easier. Do this if necessary at first, but strive to break this habit eventually.

The more you extend your knees, the harder this exercise. For Knee Raises, try to maintain a 90 degree bend.

Try to keep your lower back on the ground throughout the exercise. Depending on your body shape, this may be difficult or impossible. However, maintain the intent to touch your lower back.

Film yourself and watch back between sets to check your form. A mirror is also useful.

If your lower back hurts, using a small pillow or small rolled up towel underneath your lower back is a temporary solution.

Keeping your thighs pressed together may help you focus on the movement.

# PROGRESSION & REGRESSION

**To make this exercise harder:** Straightening your knee a bit will make this exercise more difficult.

**To make this exercise easier:** Bending your knee more will make this exercise easier. If you are unable to do this at all, raising and descending one leg at a time (kind of like riding a bicycle) is an easier variation.

# ADVANCED KNEE RAISES

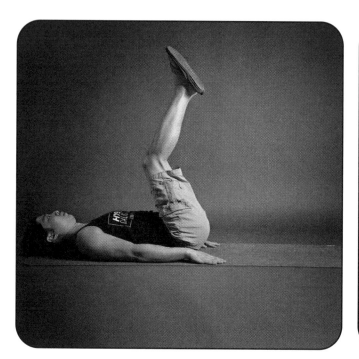

**ASCEND**

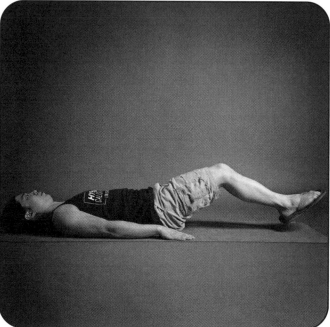

**DESCEND**

## TUTORIAL

1. Lie flat on the floor with your arms by your side.

2. Bend your knees until they are approximately 45 degrees.

3. Bring your legs up until your knees are over your waist. Control the movement.

4. Pause for 1 Second, feeling the contraction in your hips and abs.

5. Slowly descend, maintaining the 45 degree bend until your heels at 1 inch off the ground.

6. Pause for 1 Second.

7. Repeat 3-6.

## STANDARDS

**LEVEL 1:** 2 sets of 10
**LEVEL 2:** 2 sets of 20
**LEVEL 3:** 2 sets of 30

Do 2-3 sets of as many as you can.

Once you can meet or exceed Level 3 with **GOOD FORM,** you are ready to move on to a harder variation.

## BEHIND THE EXERCISE

This exercise works identically to Knee Raises. The straighter legs make the exercise harder. This continues to build a strong, powerful foundation for our waist and hips.

Aim to bend your knees around 45 degrees.

These were formerly called Bent Leg Raises.

## FORM CUES

Keep your heels off the ground throughout the exercise, Touching the ground at the bottom of the movement makes this exercise easier. Do this if necessary at first, but strive to break this habit eventually.

Try to maintain a 45 degree bend.

Try to touch your lower back to the ground as your legs go up. This strengthens our waist flexion. Depending on your body shape, this may be difficult or impossible. However, maintain the intent to touch your lower back.

Film yourself and watch back between sets to check your form. A mirror is also useful.

If your lower back hurts, using a small pillow or small rolled up towel underneath your lower back is a temporary solution.

Keeping your thighs pressed together may help you focus on the movement.

## PROGRESSION & REGRESSION

**To make this exercise harder:** Straightening your knees a bit will make this exercise more difficult.

**To make this exercise easier:** Bending your knees more will make this exercise easier, descending one leg at a time (kind of like riding a bicycle) is an easier variation.

# ALTERNATING LEG RAISES

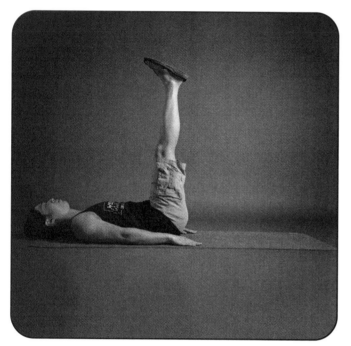

**ASCEND**

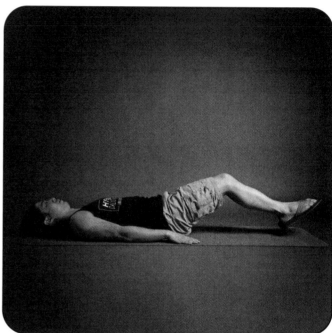

**DESCEND**

## TUTORIAL

1. Lie flat on the floor with your arms by your side.

2. Bend your knees until they are approximately 45 degrees.

3. Bring your legs up until your knees are over your waist. Control the movement.

4. Straighten at the knees.

5. Pause for 1 Second, feeling the contraction in your hips and abs.

6. Slowly descend, maintaining straight legs until your heels are 1 inch off the ground.

7. Pause for 1 Second.

8. Repeat 3-6.

## STANDARDS

**LEVEL 1:** 2 sets of 10
**LEVEL 2:** 2 sets of 15
**LEVEL 3:** 2 sets of 25

Do 2-3 sets of as many as you can.

Once you can meet or exceed Level 3 with **GOOD FORM,** you are ready to move on to a harder variation.

# BEHIND THE EXERCISE

This step helps build the strength-flexibility necessary to do good Leg Raises!

We raise our legs with our knees bent at 45 degrees, straighten our legs at the top, and descend with straight legs.

We are always able to lower a heavier weight than we can lift. The alternating nature of this exercise increases the difficulty of the negative portion - allowing us to build strength while exploring new mobility standards.

# FORM CUES

Keep your heels off the ground throughout the exercise, Touching the ground at the bottom of the movement makes this exercise easier. Do this if necessary at first, but strive to break this habit eventually.

At the top of the movement, straighten your legs, push them up, and try to touch your lower back. This increases waist activation.

Film yourself and watch back between sets to check your form. A mirror is also useful.

If your lower back hurts, using a small pillow or small rolled up towel underneath your lower back is a temporary solution.

Keeping your thighs pressed together may help you focus on the movement.

# PROGRESSION & REGRESSION

**To make this exercise harder:** Straightening the legs slightly on the way up will increase the difficulty of this exercise. If you do this slowly over time, you'll naturally be doing the next step – Leg Raises!

**To make this exercise easier:** Maintaining a slight bend at the knees will make this exercise easier. Straighten over time.

# FULL LEG RAISES

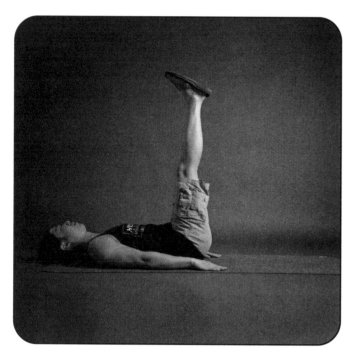

**ASCEND**

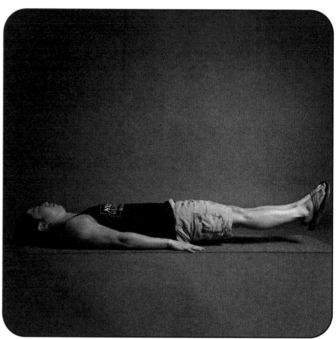

**DESCEND**

## TUTORIAL

1. Lie flat on the floor with your arms by your side.

2. Maintaining straight legs, bring your legs up until your knees are over your waist. Control the movement.

3. Pause for 1 Second, feeling the contraction in your hips and abs.

4. Slowly descend, maintaining straight legs until your heels are 1 inch off the ground.

5. Pause for 1 Second.

6. Repeat 3-5.

# STANDARDS

**LEVEL 1:** 2 sets of 5
**LEVEL 2:** 2 sets of 15
**LEVEL 3:** 2 sets of 25

Do 2-3 sets of as many as you can.

Once you can meet or exceed Level 3 with **GOOD FORM,** you are ready to move on to a harder variation.

# BEHIND THE EXERCISE

This calisthenics standard has been around for a long time. It's easy to see why. It's about as simple as a movement could get, yet builds solid strength and muscle in our waist and hips.

Although commonly overlooked for it's cousin – the Sit up – Leg Raises are generally more difficult and scalable. This means we can get more out of it!

Don't be focused on "feeling the burn" in your abs. You don't burn off fat in that way. Fat loss happens throughout our body largely through diet and exercise. If you want defined abs, build up muscle with Leg Raise progressions first. Then adjust your diet to reduce your body fat percentage until your abs show.

Maintaining fully straight legs up and down is already a challenge, but the standard for this exercise brings our legs further than usual. This starts building the lower back mobility necessary for the harder exercises!

# FORM CUES

Keep your heels off the ground throughout the exercise, Touching the ground at the bottom of the movement makes this exercise easier. Do this if necessary at first, but strive to break this habit eventually.

Like the previous step, you may have trouble straightening your legs at first. Work on this over time.

Pointing your toes will make this exercise look slightly nicer and decrease hamstring flexibility requirements. However, aim to be able to do this regardless of your ankle position.

Film yourself and watch back between sets to check your form. A mirror is also useful.

If your lower back hurts, using a small pillow or small rolled up towel underneath your lower back is a temporary solution.

Keeping your thighs pressed together may help you focus on the movement.

# PROGRESSION & REGRESSION

**To make this exercise harder:** Moving our legs beyond perpendicular to the ground will make this exercise more difficult. This is what we'll explore in our next progression!

**To make this exercise easier:** Maintaining a slight bend at the knees will make this exercise easier. Straighten over time. Doing this faster will also make it easier. Slow down over time. We want control over every part of our range of motion.

# TUCK PLOW RAISES

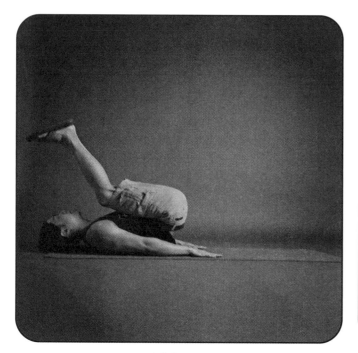

**ASCEND**

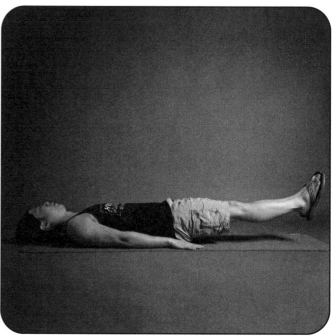

**DESCEND**

## TUTORIAL

1. Lie flat on the floor with your arms by your side.

2. Smoothly bend your knees while bringing your legs up until your thighs are firmly pressed against your chest. Your lower back should be slightly off the ground.

3. Pause for 2-3 Seconds, trying to press your thighs as firmly as safely possible against your chest.

4. Slowly descend, gradually straightening your legs until your heels are 1 inch above the ground.

5. Pause for 1 Second.

6. Repeat 2-5.

## STANDARDS

**LEVEL 1:** 2 sets of 10
**LEVEL 2:** 2 sets of 15
**LEVEL 3:** 2 sets of 25

Do 2-3 sets of as many as you can.

Once you can meet or exceed Level 3 with **GOOD FORM,** you are ready to move on to a harder variation.

# BEHIND THE EXERCISE

The previous steps worked to establish the fundamental strength and mobility needed for Leg Raises. This can keep your core healthy and strong for years to come.

This next step begins our work towards a deeper range of motion - bring the legs all the way over our body.

Because the legs are not fully extended, this gradually introduces the core strength and lower back flexibility necessary for full Plow Raises.

# FORM CUES

You may have trouble getting your waist to flex this far. Think of this as a "strength stretch." Spend a few seconds at the top trying to press your thighs firmly against your chest. Combine this with some lower back stretches will give you the necessary mobility over time. Progressive Jefferson Curls or Elephant Walks work well.

If this exercise causes cramping, take a few moments to relax and stretch before revisiting it.

Because we are bending our knees again, the bottom part of this movement will be significantly easier than the previous step. Follow this exercise with a set of Full Leg Raises.

Don't let your heels touch at the bottom of the movement. Keep them an inch off the ground.

Film yourself and watch back between sets to check your form. A mirror is also useful.

If your lower back hurts, using a small pillow or small rolled up towel underneath your lower back is a temporary solution.

Keeping your thighs pressed together may help you focus on the movement.

# PROGRESSION & REGRESSION

**To make this exercise harder:** Keeping your legs as straight as possible throughout your range of motion will make this exercise harder and introduce you to the next step.

**To make this exercise easier:** Keeping the knees bent throughout this exercise will make it easier.

# PLOW RAISES

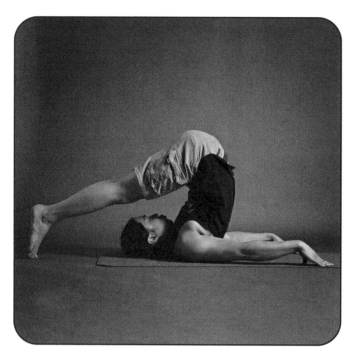

ASCEND

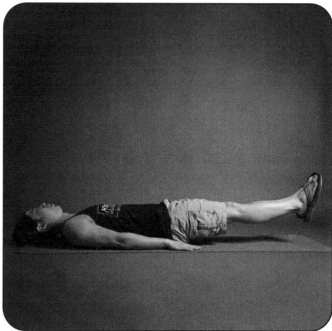

DESCEND

## TUTORIAL

1. Lie flat on the floor with your arms by your side.

2. Maintaining straight legs, smoothly bring your legs up until your toes touch the floor behind you. Your lower back should be slightly off the ground.

3. Pause for 2-3 Seconds, trying to press your thighs as firmly as safely possible against your chest.

4. Slowly descend, gradually straightening your legs until your heels are 1 inch above the ground.

5. Pause for 1 Second.

6. Repeat 2-5.

## STANDARDS

**LEVEL 1:** 2 sets of 10
**LEVEL 2:** 2 sets of 15
**LEVEL 3:** 2 sets of 25

Do 2-3 sets of as many as you can.

Once you can meet or exceed Level 3 with **GOOD FORM,** you are ready to move on to a harder variation.

# BEHIND THE EXERCISE

This is a natural continuation of Tuck Plow Raises. Maintaining straight legs retains the range of motion while increasing resistance.

The name sake of this exercise refers to the Plow Pose in yoga.

# FORM CUES

You may have trouble getting your waist to flex this far. Think of this as a "strength stretch." Spend a few seconds at the top trying to press your thighs firmly against your chest. Combine this with some lower back stretches to give you the necessary mobility over time. Progressive Jefferson Curls or Elephant Walks can work well.

It may be difficult to keep straight legs throughout the exercise. Follow this exercise with some hamstring stretches and you will eventually be able to do this!

If this exercise causes cramping, take a few moments to relax and stretch before revisiting it.

Don't let your heels touch at the bottom of the movement. Keep them an inch off the ground.

Film yourself and watch back between sets to check your form. A mirror is also useful.

Keeping your thighs pressed together may help you focus on the movement.

# PROGRESSION & REGRESSION

**To make this exercise harder:** Adding ankle weights (5-10 lb) to this exercise can make it more difficult and increase your range of motion. However, it is sufficient to meet the Level 3 standard of this exercise with perfect form before moving on to the next step.

**To make this exercise easier:** Keeping the knees bent throughout this exercise will make it easier. Keep your legs straight for as long as possible and bend as needed.

# HANGING KNEE RAISES

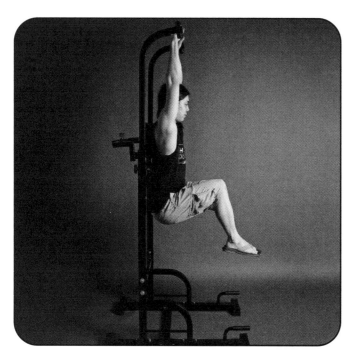

**ASCEND**

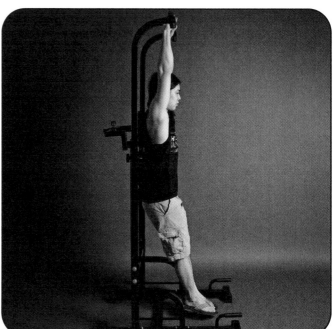

**DESCEND**

## TUTORIAL

1. Grab an overhead bar or rings with a shoulder width grip.

2. Engage your core by tilting your pelvis back.

3. Smoothly bring your legs up, simultaneously bending your knees until your thighs are parallel to the ground.

4. Pause for 1 Second.

5. Slowly reverse the movement, straightening your legs and keeping your pelvis rotated back.

6. Pause for 1 Second.

7. Repeat 3-5.

# BEHIND THE EXERCISE

Having mastered floor Leg Raises, it's time to work on doing them vertically!

Hanging knee raises may not be as difficult as Plow Raises, but they gradually introduce the grip and arm strength necessary for Hanging Leg Raises. It's a good idea to follow these with a few sets of Plow Raises.

# FORM CUES

Maintain a firm grip throughout the exercise. If you do not have the grip strength necessary for this, work just hanging from a bar until you do.

The straighter your legs, the harder this exercise is. Aim to bend your knees at 90 degrees at the top of this exercise.

You may need to bend your arms and keep your shoulders "down" to avoid pain at first. Work towards gradually straightening your arms and relaxing your shoulders for maximal core work.

Try to keep your pelvis tilted back at the bottom of the exercise. This will keep your working muscles braced throughout. While not necessary, this helps some people avoid lower back pain.

It may be tempting to forcefully bring up your knees. While there is a place for this, aim to do this exercise slowly under full control first. Then explore explosive movement as you'd like.

# PROGRESSION & REGRESSION

**To make this exercise harder:** Straightening your legs a bit will make this exercise harder and lead you smoothly into the next step!

**To make this exercise easier:** Keeping your knees bent throughout the exercise will make this easier. Take extra caution not to fall on your knees. This could seriously injure you.

# ADVANCED HANGING KNEE RAISES

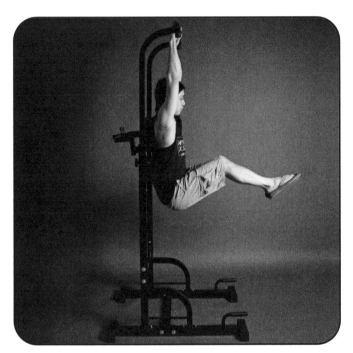

**ASCEND**

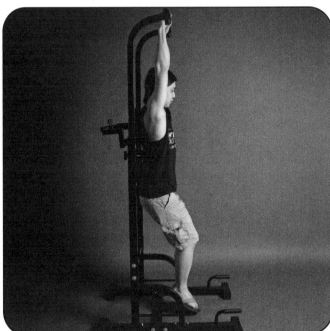

**DESCEND**

## TUTORIAL

1. Grab an overhead bar or rings with a shoulder width grip.

2. Engage your core by tilting your pelvis back.

3. Bend your knees into a 45 degree angle.

4. Smoothly bring your legs up, maintaining your knee bend until your thighs are parallel to the ground.

5. Pause for 1 Second.

6. Slowly reverse the movement, maintaining knee bend and keeping your pelvis rotated back.

7. Pause for 1 Second.

8. Repeat 4-7.

# STANDARDS

**LEVEL 1:** 2 sets of 5
**LEVEL 2:** 2 sets of 10
**LEVEL 3:** 2 sets of 15

Do 2-3 sets of as many as you can.

Once you can meet or exceed Level 3 with **GOOD FORM,** you are ready to move on to a harder variation.

# BEHIND THE EXERCISE

This exercise works almost identically to Hanging Knee Raises.

Straightening your legs makes this exercise more difficult.

To amplify this, the knee bend is retained throughout the motion.

# FORM CUES

The straighter your legs, the more difficult this exercise. Aim to maintain a 45 degree bend throughout the exercise.

Maintain a firm grip throughout the exercise. If you do not have the grip strength necessary for this, work just hanging from a bar until you do.

You may need to bend your arms and keep your shoulders "down" to avoid pain at first. Work towards gradually straightening your arms and relaxing your shoulders for maximal core work.

Try to keep your pelvis tilted back at the bottom of the exercise. This will keep your working muscles braced throughout. While not necessary, this helps some people avoid lower back pain.

It may be tempting to forcefully bring up your legs. While there is a place for this, aim to do this exercise slowly under full control first. Then explore explosive movement as you'd like.

# PROGRESSION & REGRESSION

**To make this exercise harder:** Straightening your legs a bit will make this exercise harder and lead you smoothly into the next step!

**To make this exercise easier:** Straightening your legs as you descend and bending as you ascend will make this exercise easier.

# HANGING LEG RAISES

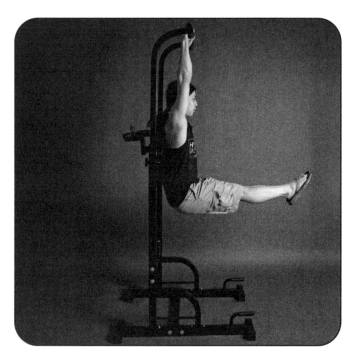

**ASCEND**

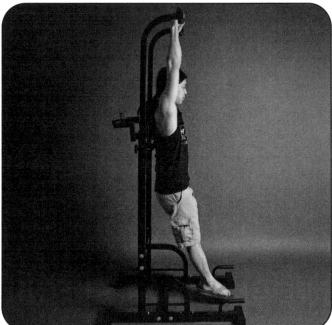

**DESCEND**

## TUTORIAL

1. Grab an overhead bar or rings with a shoulder width grip.

2. Engage your core by tilting your pelvis back.

3. Smoothly bring your legs up, keeping them perfectly straight until they are parallel to the ground.

4. Pause for 1 Second.

5. Slowly reverse the movement, keeping your pelvis rotated back.

6. Pause for 1 Second.

7. Repeat 3-6.

## STANDARDS

**LEVEL 1:** 2 sets of 10
**LEVEL 2:** 2 sets of 15
**LEVEL 3:** 2 sets of 25

Do 2-3 sets of as many as you can.

Once you can meet or exceed Level 3 with **GOOD FORM**, you are ready to move on to a harder variation.

# BEHIND THE EXERCISE

This is another calisthenics standard! Congratulations on attaining this!

This a natural continuation of the previous step. Maintaining straight legs throughout the exercise increases the difficulty.

Take some time to build up some endurance in this movement before moving on. This will help your grip strength and overall endurance.

# FORM CUES

Keep your legs straight throughout the exercise.

Maintain a firm grip throughout the exercise. If you do not have the grip strength necessary for this, work just hanging from a bar until you do.

You may need to bend your arms and keep your shoulders "down" to avoid pain at first. Work towards gradually straightening your arms and relaxing your shoulders for maximal core work.

Try to keep your pelvis tilted back at the bottom of the exercise. This will keep your working muscles braced throughout. While not necessary, this helps some people avoid lower back pain.

It may be tempting to forcefully bring up your legs. While there is a place for this, aim to do this exercise slowly under full control first. Then explore explosive movement as you'd like.

# PROGRESSION & REGRESSION

**To make this exercise harder:** Increasing the range of motion of this exercise by bringing your legs above parallel will make this exercise more difficult! Pausing in this position can even challenge some advanced athletes. This will lead you smoothly into the next step.

**To make this exercise easier:** Bending your legs on the way up and straightening on the way down will make this exercise easier.

# TOE TO BARS

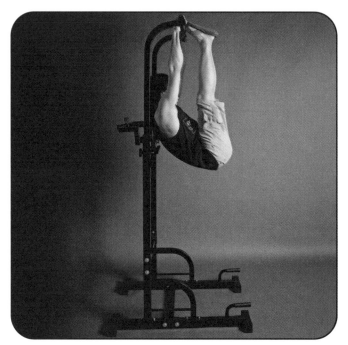

**ASCEND**

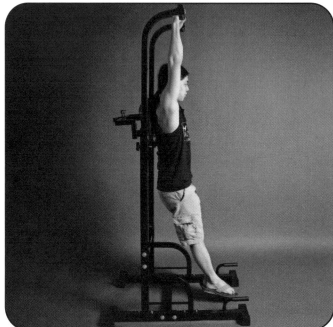

**DESCEND**

## TUTORIAL

1. Grab an overhead bar or rings with a shoulder width grip.

2. Engage your core by tilting your pelvis back.

3. Smoothly bring your legs up, keeping them perfectly straight until they touch the bar or your thighs are compressed against your chest.

4. Pause for 2-3 Seconds, firmly pressing your thighs against your chest.

5. Slowly reverse the movement, keeping your pelvis rotated back.

6. Pause for 1 Second.

7. Repeat 3-6.

# STANDARDS

**LEVEL 1:** 2 sets of 10
**LEVEL 2:** 2 sets of 15
**LEVEL 3:** 2 sets of 25

Do 2-3 sets of as many as you can.

Once you can meet or exceed Level 3 with **GOOD FORM,** you are ready to move on to a harder variation.

# BEHIND THE EXERCISE

Similar to Plow Raises, bringing our toes to touch the bar completes the range of motion.

Though you may feel the need to bend your legs at first, work on doing this with straight legs.

This strength and mobility standard is a respectable feat! Congratulations! Building up the repetitions in this movement will give you awesome core endurance and give you a head start in the other calisthenics "tricks" you may want to explore, such as Levers and Flags!

# FORM CUES

Keep your legs straight throughout the exercise.

Avoid leaning back in this exercise as much as possible. Though it may be necessary to some extent, leaning back too far will bring in your lats and decrease core work.

Do not do this exercise if your grip is failing. Falling on your lower back can paralyze you or worse.

Try to keep your pelvis tilted back at the bottom of the exercise. This will keep your working muscles braced throughout. While not necessary, this helps some people avoid lower back pain.

It may be tempting to forcefully bring up your legs. While there is a place for this, aim to do this exercise slowly under full control first. Then explore explosive movement as you'd like.

# PROGRESSION & REGRESSION

**To make this exercise harder:** Exploring gymnastic holds like the V-Sit, I-Sit, and Manna can take your midsection work to the next level!

**To make this exercise easier:** Bending your knees as necessary will make this exercise easier.

# CLOSING THOUGHTS

That concludes the Leg Raise series! If you have mastered all of the variations in the series, you've built a strong and stable core. Congratulations!

Take notice of all the ways a strong core plays a role in your life. Activities like picking up a hefty cat, putting luggage in an overhead bin, or kayaking on a river require a solid and stable core. You'll also benefit from your strong hip flexors any time you go for a walk, run, hike, or bike ride!

So, where do you go from here? That's a great question because there are endless ways to challenge your core strength! You will never run out of things to try. Here are some variations to give you a starting point:

**L Sit** - This isometric exercise is a great way to continue to challenge and strengthen your lower abdominals. You can do this on parallel bars or in a sturdy chair.

Another version of this exercise is a V Sit! You can probably imagine what that looks like compared to an L Sit. Instead of holding your legs out at a 90-degree angle, you'll raise them up to about 45 degrees and hold your position there!

Both of these variations can also be done while hanging from a pullup bar or gym rings! Just remember to breathe as you hold the position.

**Clutch Flag / Human Flag** - This exercise is simply iconic in the world of calisthenics. Now that you have developed excellent core strength, it will be easier to get the hang of this impressive exercise.

Note that I said easier, not easy! This exercise will challenge your obliques in a way that the leg raise series did not. You will still have a challenge ahead of you!

**Suspension Pikes** - You've got strong hip flexors and a stable core, so it might be time to add an element of instability! If you have gym rings, you can lower them until they are approximately one foot above the floor. You will start in a plank position with your feet in the rings, suspended off the ground. When you go into your pike position, your core will work extra hard to minimize any wobbling!

---

A lot of people will only do Leg Raises to "get abs." While they're highly effective for this purpose, Leg Raises also build a functional and strong midsection to your body. You may have noticed that this area gets worked in almost all exercises. This translates well to real life, where our midsection is used in almost everything we do! Your body will thank you for giving this area some extra love.

## Where do I start?

Start with a variation that you can do competently with good form for at least a few repetitions. When in doubt, start with Knee Raises!

## This exercise feels uncomfortable in my lower back. How do I fix this?

It could be that your pelvis is tipping forward during your leg raises. Before you begin, imagine scooping your tailbone to the sky. This should help you maintain a neutral pelvis.

Alternatively, you can simply do each exercise as an isometric hold. Instead of raising and lowering your legs, you can simply raise your legs and keep them there - different positions will have varying difficulty. This applies to any exercise, but especially to Leg Raises. The primary muscles involved are often used for stability anyway.

However, it's always a good idea to check in with your doctor or physical therapist when you start experiencing new or worsening pain. Addressing issues early on can save you from a lot more pain later in life.

## I have met the standard for one variation, but the next exercise feels too hard. What should I do?

Each exercise has a Progression and a Regression. You can use these to your advantage!

Let's say you are stuck somewhere between two exercises. When it comes to Leg Raise variations, you can make the exercise easier or harder by bending or straightening your legs a little more.

The Progression (straighter legs) will challenge your body in preparation for the next exercise. The Regression (slightly more bent legs) will allow you to ease into the full exercise.

You can think of these as transition exercises!

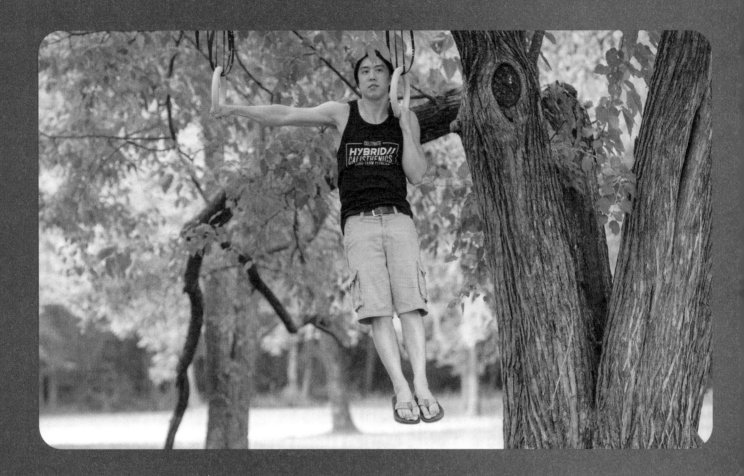

# PULLUPS

The Pullup is another classic movement that comes to mind when we think about exercise. In fact, pulling is another one of our most fundamental movement patterns! Think of pulling out a chair, pulling your garage door shut, or reigning in your dog's leash when they want to chase a squirrel. The pulling movement pattern happens daily!

As we know, Pullups aren't easy. Many of us have never been able to do a Full Pullup with good form before, let alone a One-

Arm Pullup! That's why we put together this selection of progressions. Start where you are and build up your strength with a healthy movement pattern.

Every variation on a Pullup is a compound movement that works a large muscle group. In the pulling or concentric phase, this exercise utilizes our latissimus dorsi, posterior deltoids, trapezius, and biceps. A number of stabilizing muscles are working throughout the entire movement.

# GENERAL PULLUP CUES

Allow your shoulder blades to move naturally. Retract them at the top and protract them at the bottom.

Video yourself and watch back between sets to monitor your form!

It's common to refer an overhand grip as Pullups and an underhand grip as Chinups. Overhand will have more emphasis on the back and underhand will have more emphasis on the biceps. They are comparable in difficulty. Aim to master both, as well as a neutral grip (thumbs facing back)!

"Perfect form" for Pullups is often debated. You'll get different answers depending on who you ask. As long as you build up to your technique progressively (without sudden increases in resistance), you should be safe. Aim be able to do all of them!

# PULLUP PROGRESSIONS

First, we start by introducing our bodies to the pulling movement pattern at a less intense angle. When we do a pulling exercise from a less severe angle, we can concentrate on getting the movement down before moving on to a more demanding variation. The closer we are to the ground, the more strength is required!

After we have mastered the first three variations, we can start locking in good form with Jackknife Pullups. We'll gradually reduce the need for assistance and graduate to the world of Full Pullups! Once we have mastered Narrow Pullups, we'll start exploring the single-arm variations for this exercise. There are several exercise variations here to help your body transition to this new challenge. Taking the time to master these variations will help strengthen and protect your joints - it's a worthwhile endeavor!

Let's get to pulling!

1. Wall Pullups
2. Horizontal Pullups
3. Advanced Incline Pullups
4. Jackknife Pullups
5. Full Pullups
6. Narrow Pullups
7. One-Hand Pullups
8. Advanced One-Hand Pullups
9. Archer Pullups
10. One-Arm Pullups

# WALL PULLUPS

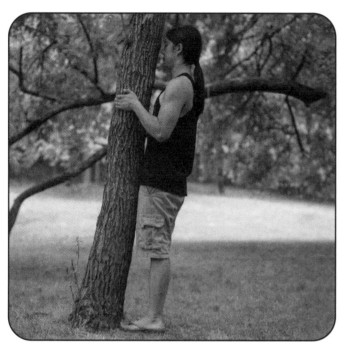

**ASCEND**

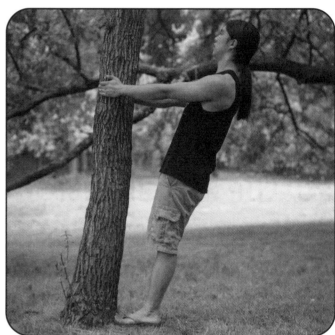

**DESCEND**

## TUTORIAL

1. Stand at arm's length facing a pole, tree, or wall section.

2. Firmly grasp the object with both arms. Your arms should be straight.

3. Ascend slowly until the object or your hands gently touch your chest.

4. Pause for 1 Second.

5. Slowly come back down.

6. Pause for 1 Second.

7. Repeat 3-6.

# STANDARDS

**LEVEL 1:** 2 sets of 30
**LEVEL 2:** 2 sets of 50
**LEVEL 3:** 3 sets of 50

Do 2-3 sets of as many as you can.

Once you can meet or exceed Level 3 with **GOOD FORM,** you are ready to move on to a harder variation.

# BEHIND THE EXERCISE

Vertical pulling is one of the gentlest ways to introduce pulling with a full range of motion.

The high angle makes this movement a lot easier than Horizontal or Full Pullups.

Although these may feel very easy, it's useful to practice these for a few weeks to feel how your joints want move and build healthy movement patterns.

They're also a great therapy exercise. The gentle movement stretches stiff muscles and heals old wounds.

Keep your shoulder blades down and back to better engage your back muscles. Learning to do this with straight arms at the bottom of the movement will build fundamental scapular strength - very important for advanced calisthenics!

# FORM CUES

The higher the base you grasp - the easier this exercise. For this step, find something around sternum height.

Try to maintain a consistent height so you can better judge your progress. Small adjustments over time are fine!

This is where having a set of Gymnastic Rings really shines. They'll allow you to pull higher. If using a bar, pull until your chest touches the bar. If using rings, pull until your fists are by your chest.

Keep your body firm. Don't arch your body at the bottom to make the motion easier. Core strength is important for all calisthenics, and this is a great place to start building it.

# PROGRESSION & REGRESSION

**To make this exercise harder:** Doing this with one-arm is doable even for some beginners and offers an interesting change.

**To make this exercise easier:** Finding an object you can grasp firmly will make this exercise safer and more effective. This exercise should not be much harder than opening a heavy door.

# HORIZONTAL PULLUPS

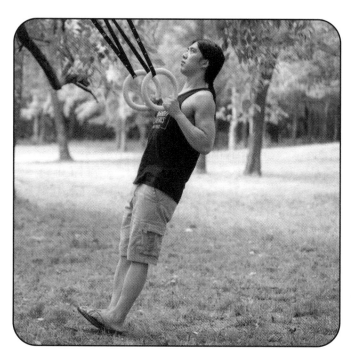

**ASCEND**

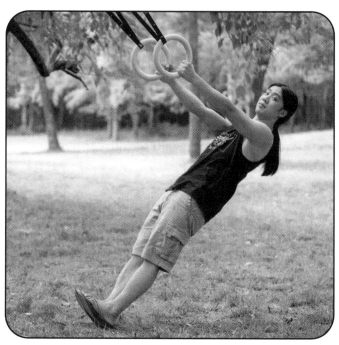

**DESCEND**

## TUTORIAL

1. Get below a horizontal base that is sternum height when you're standing.

2. Firmly grasp the base with both arms at shoulder width. Your arms should be straight.

3. Ascend slowly until the base or your hands gently touch your chest.

4. Pause for 1 Second.

5. Slowly come back down.

6. Pause for 1 Second.

7. Repeat 3-6.

## STANDARDS

**LEVEL 1:** 2 sets of 15
**LEVEL 2:** 2 sets of 30
**LEVEL 3:** 3 sets of 30

Do 2-3 sets of as many as you can.

Once you can meet or exceed Level 3 with **GOOD FORM,** you are ready to move on to a harder variation.

# BEHIND THE EXERCISE

With the previous exercise, there was little or no tension at the top of the exercise - the user was simply standing.

With this, we begin training strength throughout our entire exercise set!

While not as difficult as Full Pullups, these exercise train horizontal pulling - a very important fundamental movement.

Find a base around sternum height for this step. The high angle makes this easy enough for focus on form while offering enough intensity to build some strength and muscle!

# FORM CUES

Slow and steady wins the race on this exercise. Don't just speed through these. Find a controlled, rhythmic pace to really feel this movement. 2 Seconds Down, 1 Second Pause, 2 Seconds Up. Repeat.

Keep your hands around sternum height. Your fist should touch your chest at the top of the movement.

Regardless of where you do this exercise, make sure you have a good grip on the object. A slippery surface will make holding on difficult, which is not the goal of this exercise.

Keep your body firm. Don't arch your body at the bottom to make the motion easier. Core strength is important for all calisthenics, and this is a great place to start building it.

# PROGRESSION & REGRESSION

**To make this exercise harder:** Using a lower base will make this exercise more difficult and lead naturally to the next progression!

**To make this exercise easier:** A higher base will make this exercise easier. Alternatively, you can bend your knees a bit!

# ADVANCED HORIZONTAL PULLUPS

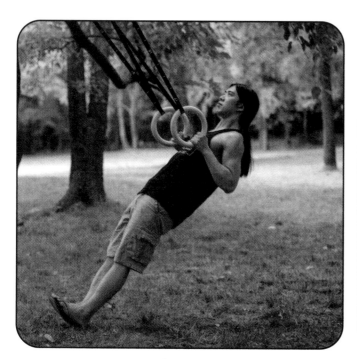

**ASCEND**

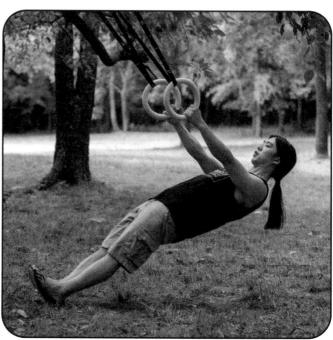

**DESCEND**

## TUTORIAL

1. Get below a horizontal base that is hip height when you're standing.

2. Firmly grasp the base with both arms at shoulder width. Your arms should be straight.

3. Ascend slowly until the base or your hands gently touch your chest.

4. Pause for 1 Second.

5. Slowly come back down.

6. Pause for 1 Second.

7. Repeat 3-6.

# STANDARDS

**LEVEL 1:** 2 sets of 10
**LEVEL 2:** 2 sets of 15
**LEVEL 3:** 3 sets of 25

Do 2–3 sets of as many as you can.

Once you can meet or exceed Level 3 with **GOOD FORM,** you are ready to move on to a harder variation.

# BEHIND THE EXERCISE

This is a simple continuation of Horizontal Pullups.

The movement is the same, but the lower base will make this exercise harder.

Aim to do this with a base at hip height.

# FORM CUES

Start filming yourself around this step. Watch back between sets to monitor your form! This applies to many exercises.

The higher the base you grasp – the easier this exercise. For this step, find something around hip height.

Try to maintain a consistent height so you can better judge your progress. Small adjustments over time are fine!

Keep your body firm. Don't arch your body at the bottom to make the motion easier. Core strength is important for all calisthenics, and this is a great place to start building it.

# PROGRESSION & REGRESSION

**To make this exercise harder:** Using a lower base will make this exercise more difficult. Alternatively, you can bend at the hips and pull vertically. This will be very similar to the next progression!

**To make this exercise easier:** A higher base will make this exercise easier. Alternatively, you can bend your knees a bit!

# JACKKNIFE PULLUPS

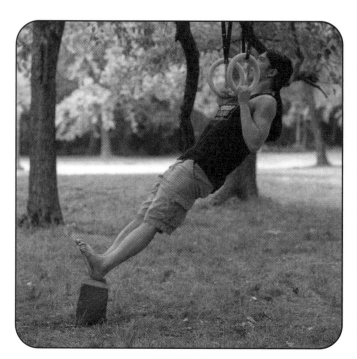

**ASCEND**

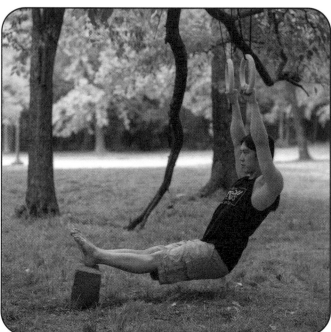

**DESCEND**

## TUTORIAL

1. Sit below a horizontal base with your legs straight in front of you.

2. Firmly grasp the base with both arms at shoulder width. Your arms should be straight and your butt off the ground.

3. Ascend slowly until the base or your hands gently touch your chest. Assist with your legs as necessary.

4. Pause for 1 Second.

5. Slowly come back down.

6. Pause for 1 Second.

7. Repeat 3-6.

## STANDARDS

**LEVEL 1:** 2 sets of 5
**LEVEL 2:** 2 sets of 15
**LEVEL 3:** 3 sets of 20

Do 2-3 sets of as many as you can.

Once you can meet or exceed Level 3 with **GOOD FORM,** you are ready to move on to a harder variation.

# BEHIND THE EXERCISE

After developing our strength in horizontal pulling, we're ready to explore assisted vertical pulling.

Vertical pulling can be more difficult - so we assist with our legs!

It can be wise to retain horizontal pulling because it emphasizes different muscle groups. Warm up with a few sets or Horizontal Pullups - or finish up with them!

# FORM CUES

Positioning is key for Jackknife Pullups. Your torso should be slightly behind the bar. You should be able to pull your chin above the rings or bar. If you feel like your legs are "too short" to assist at the top, move your body back a bit.

Similarly, find an ideal height for the base or rings. Your butt should be an inch or so off the ground while maintaining straight arms at the bottom.

At first, your torso will start off vertical and lean back as you go up. Over time, try to maintain a somewhat vertical torso as you ascend.

This is where having a set of Gymnastic Rings really shines. They'll allow you to pull higher. If using a bar, pull until your chest touches the bar. If using rings, pull until your fists are by your chest.

While you will need to hinge at the hips for this exercise, maintain tension in your core and legs. Avoid sagging!

# PROGRESSION & REGRESSION

**To make this exercise harder:** Putting your feet on a raised base like a stool will make this exercise harder. However, this will better simulate a Full Pullup!

**To make this exercise easier:** Starting with your torso vertical and leaning back on the way up will make this exercise easier. This is essentially combining Jackknife Pullups and Horizontal Pullups.

# FULL PULLUPS

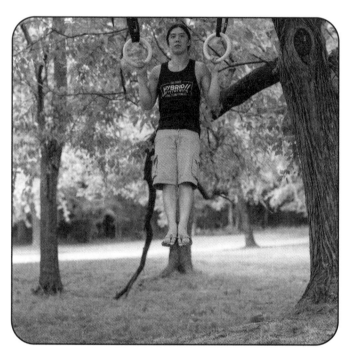

**ASCEND**

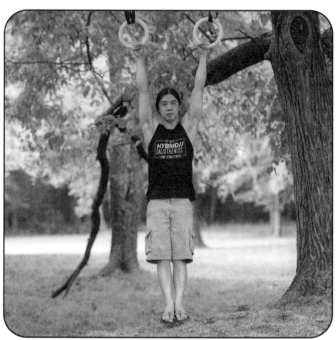

**DESCEND**

## TUTORIAL

1.  Stand below a horizontal bar or rings.

2.  Firmly grasp the bar with both arms at shoulder width. Your entire body should be straight and off the ground.

3.  Ascend slowly until your chest gently touches the bar (or just below).

4.  Pause for 1 Second.

5.  Slowly come back down.

6.  Pause for 1 Second.

7.  Repeat 3-6.

# STANDARDS

**LEVEL 1:** 2 sets of 3
**LEVEL 2:** 2 sets of 6
**LEVEL 3:** 3 sets of 12

Do 2-3 sets of as many as you can.

Once you can meet or exceed Level 3 with **GOOD FORM,** you are ready to move on to a harder variation.

# BEHIND THE EXERCISE

This is another calisthenics standard! This is one of the most functional fitness movements. Period.

Congratulations if you make it here!

It's worthwhile to build up your reps in this exercise - even beyond the Level 3 standards below. This can improve your quality of life and survival ability. Humans have tremendous climbing ability - a potential that's largely untapped because of the luxuries of modern living. Reconnect with this fundamental movement and reap the benefits!

# FORM CUES

"Perfect form" for Full Pullups is often debated. You'll get different answers depending on who you ask. As long as you build up to your technique progressively (without sudden increases in resistance), you should be safe. Aim to be able to do all of them!

It's common to refer to an overhand grip as Pullups and an underhand grip as Chin ups. They emphasize slightly different muscles. They are comparable in difficulty. Aim to master both, as well as a neutral grip (thumbs facing back)!

Having Gymnastic Rings here will allow your hands to rotate freely as you do this exercise.

Video yourself and watch back between sets to monitor your form!

# PROGRESSION & REGRESSION

**To make this exercise harder:** Explore different grip positions before making the exercise more difficult. This will build a better foundation for your Pullups. Afterwards, experiment with bringing your hands closer together. This will increase difficulty and build the strength necessary for the next step!

**To make this exercise easier:** Using momentum from your arms or legs will make this exercise easier - sometimes referred to as "kipping." While this makes the exercise easier, the sudden forces may injure you if you're unprepared for the load. If you can do Level 3 of Jackknife Pullups but are unable to do Level 1 of Full Pullups, experiment with "negatives" by slowly lowering yourself from the top position. Alternatively, explore isometric holds at the middle and top positions.

# NARROW PULLUPS

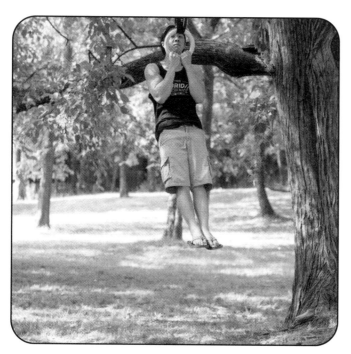

**ASCEND**

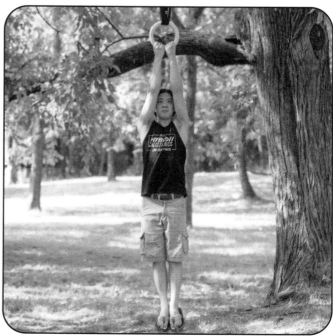

**DESCEND**

## TUTORIAL

1. Stand below a horizontal bar or rings.

2. Firmly grasp the bar with both hands. Your hands should be together. Your entire body should be straight and off the ground.

3. Ascend slowly until your chest gently touches your hands.

4. Pause for 1 Second.

5. Slowly come back down.

6. Pause for 1 Second.

7. Repeat 3-6.

# STANDARDS

**LEVEL 1:** 2 sets of 3
**LEVEL 2:** 2 sets of 6
**LEVEL 3:** 3 sets of 9

Do 2-3 sets of as many as you can.

Once you can meet or exceed Level 3 with **GOOD FORM,** you are ready to move on to a harder variation.

# BEHIND THE EXERCISE

After building fundamental vertical pulling strength with Full Pullups - we can explore using a narrow grip.

Compared to our biceps, the muscles in our back are much larger and stronger.

The narrow positioning of our hands makes it harder for them to assist. This makes our arms work harder and get much stronger as a result!

Remember a chain is only as strong as its weakest link. In any exercise, you can only lift as much as your weakest body part will allow.

Strengthening our biceps and elbow joint here will prepare us for the rigors of the next exercises!

# FORM CUES

It is usually more comfortable to do this exercise with an underhand or neutral grip.

"Perfect form" for Pullups is often debated. You'll get different answers depending on who you ask. As long as you build up to your technique progressively (without sudden increases in resistance), you should be safe. Aim be able to do all of them!

If you are using Gymnastic Rings, you may be able to do this on one ring. Make sure the single ring can support your weight!

Video yourself and watch back between sets to monitor your form!

# PROGRESSION & REGRESSION

**To make this exercise harder:** Overlapping your hands can make this exercise more difficult. Having one hand on the other can increase grip strength demands and be a good intermediary step between this and the next step. However, depending on your weight, it may leave bruises on your hand. If this happens, work up to overlapping your hands gently. This will be harder but will make you stronger!

**To make this exercise easier:** Keeping your hands further apart will make this exercise easier. If you're building up from Full Pullups, it might help to move your hands a few inches closer together every week or so. Do this if you experience joint pain! Our joints can be stronger than our muscles, but they develop more slowly.

# ONE HAND PULLUPS

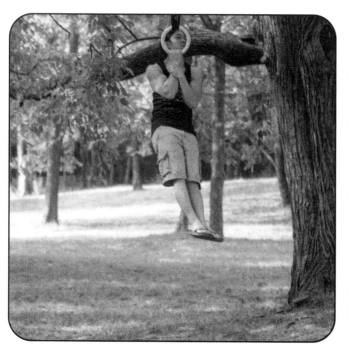

**ASCEND**

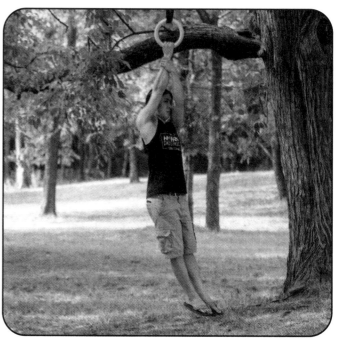

**DESCEND**

## TUTORIAL

1.   Stand below a horizontal bar or rings.

2.   Firmly grasp the bar with one hand. Use your other hand and placing it on your the wrist of your working arm.

3.   Ascend slowly until your chest gently touches your hand.

4.   Pause for 1 Second.

5.   Slowly come back down.

6.   Pause for 1 Second.

7.   Repeat 3-6.

## STANDARDS

**LEVEL 1:** 2 Sets of 3 (Both Sides)
**LEVEL 2:** 2 Sets of 6 (Both Sides)
**LEVEL 3:** 2 Sets of 9 (Both Sides)

Do 2-3 sets of as many as you can.

Once you can meet or exceed Level 3 with **GOOD FORM,** you are ready to move on to a harder variation.

# BEHIND THE EXERCISE

Now that we've prepared our arms with Narrow Pullups, it's time to begin training for one-arm pulling.

Assisting with your other arm makes this movement significantly easier. One Arm Pullups are much more difficult.

However, the grip strength demands are identical, so this will give practitioners a massive boost in their grip strength. While you may be tempted to use wrist straps or something to bridge this gap, aim to be able to hold your body with one hand.

The biceps in particular get a great workout with this exercise.

The lower you grip with your supporting arm, the harder the exercise!

Start with a grip on your wrist for this progression.

# FORM CUES

The lower your supporting hand, the harder the exercise. Start with a grip on your wrist.

If your supporting hand leaves bruises on your wrist, you may be supporting too much. Over time, allow a firm grip that doesn't leave bruises. Your working arm will get stronger as a result.

As with Narrow Pullups, this exercise is usually done with an underhand grip.

If you are using Gymnastic Rings, you may be able to do this on one ring. Make sure the single ring can support your weight!

# PROGRESSION & REGRESSION

**To make this exercise harder:** Lowering your supporting hand will make this exercise harder. Your forearm is wider than your wrist and harder to grip. This will lead you to the next exercise!

**To make this exercise easier:** Supporting more with your assisting arm will make this exercise easier.

# ADVANCED ONE HAND PULLUPS

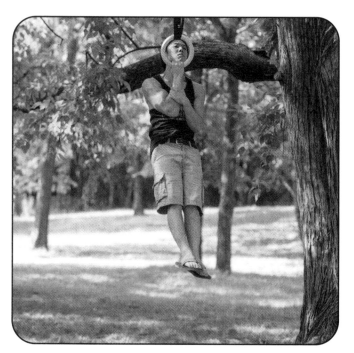

**ASCEND**

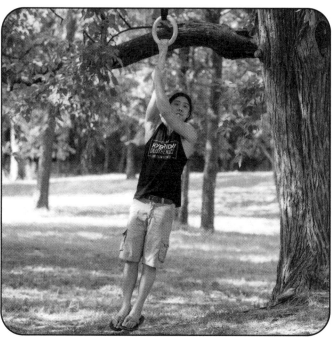

**DESCEND**

## TUTORIAL

1. Stand below a horizontal bar or rings.
2. Firmly grasp the bar with one hand. Use your other hand and placing it on the forearm of your working arm.
3. Ascend slowly until your chest gently touches your hand.
4. Pause for 1 Second.
5. Slowly come back down.
6. Pause for 1 Second.
7. Repeat 3-6.

# STANDARDS

**LEVEL 1:** 2 Sets of 3 (Both Sides)
**LEVEL 2:** 2 Sets of 6 (Both Sides)
**LEVEL 3:** 2 Sets of 9 (Both Sides)

Do 2-3 sets of as many as you can.

Once you can meet or exceed Level 3 with **GOOD FORM,** you are ready to move on to a harder variation.

## BEHIND THE EXERCISE

This is a natural progression from regular One-Hand Pullups.

Gripping at the working arm at the forearm instead of the wrist makes this exercise more difficult. Don't be surprised if your reps drop! This means your working arm has to work harder and will get stronger as a result!

## FORM CUES

The less you assist with your supporting arm, the harder this exercise will be. Start by gripping firmly and start softening your grip as you approach Level 3 of this exercise. You'll know you're almost ready to move on when you feel like you can do this exercise assisting with only a flat palm!

If your supporting hand leaves bruises on your forearm, you may be supporting too much. Over time, allow a firm grip that doesn't leave bruises. Your working arm will get stronger as a result.

As with Narrow Pullups, this exercise is usually done with an underhand grip.

If you are using Gymnastic Rings, you may be able to do this on one ring. Make sure the single ring can support your weight!

## PROGRESSION & REGRESSION

**To make this exercise harder:** Supporting less with your assisting arm will make this exercise harder. A good way is to loosen your grip overtime. When you're able to do Level 3 of this exercise with a flat palm, you're definitely ready to move on!

**To make this exercise easier:** Supporting more with your assisting arm will make this exercise easier.

# ARCHER PULLUPS

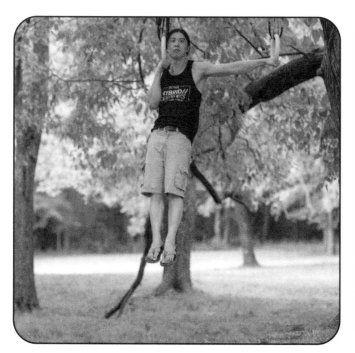

**ASCEND**

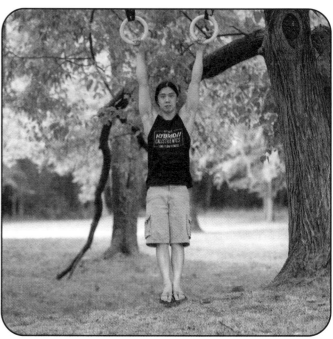

**DESCEND**

## TUTORIAL

1. Stand below a horizontal bar or rings.

2. Firmly grasp the bar with both hands. Your hands should be around twice shoulder width. Your arms should be relatively straight.

3. Ascend slowly with one arm until your chest gently touches your hand.

4. Pause for 1 Second.

5. Slowly come back down.

6. Pause for 1 Second.

7. Repeat 3-6.

## STANDARDS

**LEVEL 1:** 2 Sets of 3 (Both Sides)
**LEVEL 2:** 2 Sets of 6 (Both Sides)
**LEVEL 3:** 2 Sets of 9 (Both Sides)

Do 2-3 sets of as many as you can.

Once you can meet or exceed Level 3 with **GOOD FORM,** you are ready to move on to a harder variation.

# BEHIND THE EXERCISE

While comparable in difficulty to Advanced One-Hand Pullups, this puts different forces on our body and helps drill the movement pulling with one arm.

While the grip strength demands are not as high, the shoulders get a great workout.

It's a great idea to do 1-2 sets of Isometric One-Arm Pullups before this exercise. Holding experiment with holding the top, middle, and bottom position of the exercise for time, even if it's only a few seconds at first.

# FORM CUES

The straighter your assisting arm, the more difficult this exercise. You may find it difficult to have a completely straight arm at first. Use a slightly bent arm at first if necessary. Straighten over time.

Grip position is up to the preferences of the user. If you build the previous exercises with an underhand grip, it's a good idea to use a mixed grip - underhand with your working arm and overhand with your assisting arm.

The width between your hands is slightly dependent on the proportions and mobility of the user. Twice shoulder width is a good starting point for many people.

If you are doing this exercise on Gymnastic Rings, experiment with the width between the rings. If they're too wide, the straps may slide. Slightly less than shoulder width seems to work.

# PROGRESSION & REGRESSION

**To make this exercise harder:** After mastering this exercise with straight arms, gripping your assisting hand with fewer fingers will make this exercise more difficult.

**To make this exercise easier:** Bending your supporting arm will make this exercise easier.

# ONE ARM PULLUPS

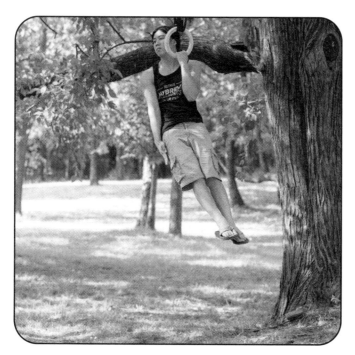

**ASCEND**

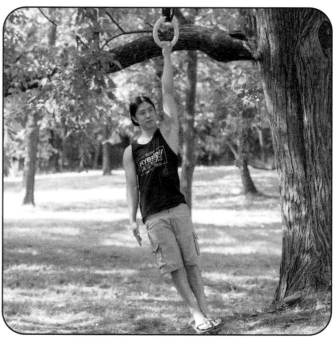

**DESCEND**

## TUTORIAL

1. Stand below a horizontal bar or rings
2. Firmly grasp the bar with one hand. Your working arm should be straight.
3. Ascend slowly until your chin is above the bar or rings. Allow your free arm to move freely for balance.
4. Pause for 1 Second.
5. Slowly come back down.
6. Pause for 1 Second.
7. Repeat 3-6.

## STANDARDS

**LEVEL 1:** 1 Set of 1 (Both Sides)
**LEVEL 2:** 2 Sets of 3 (Both Sides)
**LEVEL 3:** 2 Sets of 6 (Both Sides)

Do 2-3 sets of as many as you can.

Once you can meet or exceed Level 3 with **GOOD FORM,** you are ready to move on to a harder variation.

## BEHIND THE EXERCISE

While comparable in difficulty to Advanced One-Hand Pullups, this puts different forces on our body and helps drill the movement pulling with one arm.

While the grip strength demands are not as high, the shoulders get a great workout.

It's a great idea to do 1-2 sets of Isometric One-Arm Pullups before this exercise. Holding experiment with holding the top, middle, and bottom position of the exercise for time, even if it's only a few seconds at first.

## FORM CUES

Whatever progressions you use to build up to this step, strive to be able to do it with clean form and without joint pain. Train for strength, health, and ability - not ego!

Grip position is up to the preferences of the user. Some might find an underhand grip easier, but it appears to be dependent on the individual. Strive to master all grip types.

If you are using Gymnastic Rings, you may be able to do this on one ring. Make sure the single ring can support your weight!

## PROGRESSION & REGRESSION

**To make this exercise harder:** After mastering this exercise (congratulations!), strive to master it with all the grip positions. Then try using fewer fingers to grip. This is an endeavor that may take several years. From this point on, you can experiment with weighted pullups, both with one arm and two arms. Try new things and push the boundaries of your limits! Safely, of course. I'm very proud of you!

**To make this exercise easier:** Using partial range of motion or isometrics will make this exercise easier. For more people, the bottom part (from dead hang to engaged scapula) and the top part (chin going above the bar or rings) are the hardest. Working the range in between can help you build the strength for full range of motion.

# CLOSING THOUGHTS

This brings us to a close for the Pullup series! If you have completed the whole Pullup series, you have developed significant upper body strength and mastered a fundamental movement pattern. Time to celebrate!

While we might not be doing a lot of loaded overhead pulling outside of a dedicated workout, horizontal pulling is a recurring movement pattern day to day. We pull to open a door, start a lawn mower, and play tug-o-war with a dog. Try to count all the pulls you do in a day! It's probably more than you think.

So, what's next now that you've mastered your pullups? You can try a variety of things, from isometrics to explosive movements. Here are some variations that might be of interest:

**Monkey Bars -** Hit the playground, my friend! Your grip strength and One Arm Pullup skills will translate well to swinging from bar to bar. You'll find more challenging versions of a swinging exercise if you sign up for an obstacle course race!

**Muscle Up -** This exercise combines a pullup with a dip to create one fluid motion. You use explosive power and momentum to pull your body up past the bar, then push down into the bar to straighten your arms at the top!

This is a challenging exercise that requires good coordination and honed technique. Seeing this exercise performed often elicits a "wow" from bystanders. Make sure you have truly mastered the Full Pullup (at least) before trying this exercise! Having a spotter with you is also a good idea.

**One Arm Horizontal Pullups -** Some analytical readers might have observed that our Pullup series begins with horizontal pulling and gradually transitions to vertical pulling. Doing this builds strength and skill in both valuable movements. Because of how we've structured this series, the vertical pulling variations are inherently more difficult.

That doesn't mean we have to forget horizontal pulling, though! Similar to how we transitioned from Full Pullups to Narrow Pullups, we can do the same with Narrow Horizontal Pullups! From there, assistance can be used to gradually transition to one-arm horizontal pulling. This emphasizes slightly different muscles from their vertical counterparts. Aim to master both! This can also be helpful for reducing muscle imbalance.

---

Swinging from bars and climbing trees came naturally to some of us as children. As we grow older, we often lose these habits. While not everyone can climb trees daily, retaining some Pullup work will keep our grip and pulling muscles healthy and strong!

### Where do I start?

Start with a variation that you can do competently with good form for at least a few repetitions. When in doubt, start with Wall Pullups!

### I don't have a place to attach gym rings or install a pullup bar. What are my options?

It's tough to replace the Full Pullup with a different bodyweight exercise. You can try using a sturdy table or a pair of sturdy chairs to do horizontal pullups, or inverted rows. These exercises will target the muscle group in a similar manner.

However, it's well worth it to find something you can use for Full Pullups. Check out your local park and see if there are some monkey bars around!

### I have met the standard for one variation, but the next exercise feels too hard. What should I do?

Each exercise has a Progression and a Regression. You can use these to your advantage!
For example, let's say you are stuck somewhere between two exercises. If your Wall Pullups are too easy, the Progression will challenge your body in preparation for the next exercise (using only one arm).

Alternatively, if the Horizontal Pullups are too challenging, the Regression will allow you to build into them more slowly (use a higher base, or bend your knees slightly).

You can think of these as transition exercises!

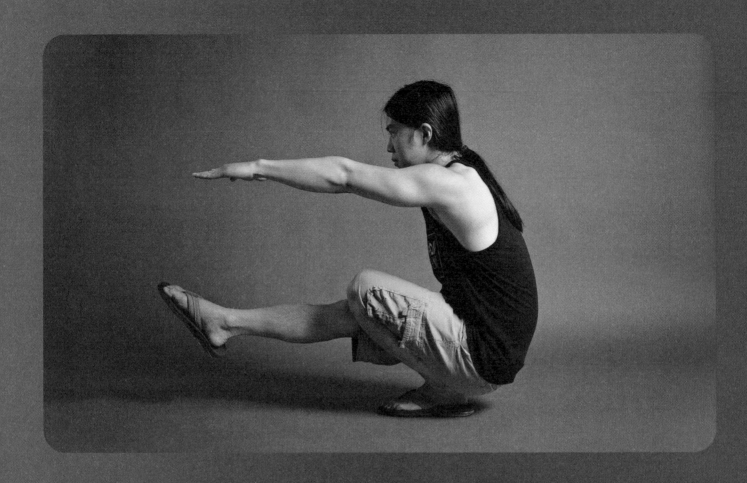

# SQUATS

The Squat is one of the most common fundamental movements we make day-to-day. Think standing up from a chair, getting up off of the ground, or even climbing a flight of stairs. We are constantly doing different variations on a Squat!

Having a great Squat pattern is a very valuable life skill. That's why we put together this selection of progressions. Start where you are and build up your strength with a healthy movement pattern.

Every variation on a Squat is a compound movement that works a large muscle group. This exercise utilizes our glutes, quadriceps, hamstrings, hip flexors, and calves. A number of stabilizing muscles are working throughout the entire movement.

# GENERAL SQUAT CUES

Slow and steady wins the race on this exercise. Don't just speed through these. Find a controlled, rhythmic pace to really feel this movement. 2 Seconds Down, 1 Second Pause, 2 Seconds Up. Repeat.

Try to keep your back neutral throughout the exercise. This means don't arch or round your back. This may take some work if you're not used to it, but you should make progress over time. The lower back may round at the very bottom of the movement, which is usually fine.

Film yourself and watch back between sets!

As we are building up progressively, it is okay for your knees to go over your toes. Doing this with an exercise we can competently handle will strengthen our joints in tandem with our muscles.

On exercises that use support from your arms, use enough support to avoid bending excessively at the hips. If you find you need to bend forward a lot to squat, try supporting your arms!

# SQUAT PROGRESSIONS

First we will explore our balance and range of motion with Jackknife and Assisted Squats. Our hips, knees, and ankles will need to be familiar with this movement pattern before we go any further. Once we know and trust our squat pattern, we can begin working on functional strength and range of motion with Half Squats, Full Squats, and Narrow Squats. These will each challenge your lower body in a unique and valuable way - mastering these will set you up for success with the next variations.

After we have mastered the bilateral squats, it's time to graduate to single-leg exercises! We will gradually learn to rely on one leg to power our movements. One-Leg Squats are an impressive feat, and it's a skill well worth pursuing!

Get out there and put your glutes to work!

1. Jackknife squats
2. Assisted Squats
3. Half Squats
4. Full Squats
5. Narrow Squats
6. Side-Staggered Squats
7. Front-Staggered Squats
8. Assisted One-Leg Squats
9. One-Leg Chair Squats
10. One-Leg Squats

# JACKKNIFE SQUATS

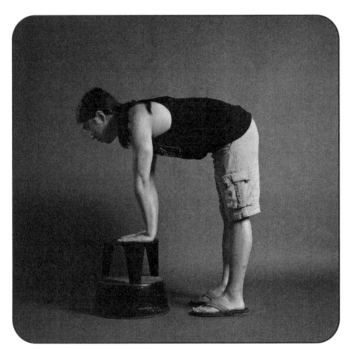

**ASCEND**

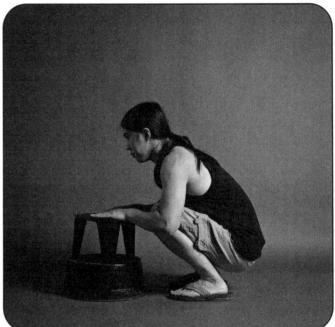

**DESCEND**

## TUTORIAL

1. Stand in front of a stable platform around knee height.

2. Maintaining straight legs, bend at the hips until your palms are on the platform. Your arms should be relatively straight, as should your waist.

3. Squat down slowly, with a slightly forward lean so you may assist with your arms, until your hamstrings are pressed against your calves. You should not be able to squat any further.

4. Pause for 1 Second.

5. Slowly come back up.

6. Pause for 1 Second.

7. Repeat 3-6.

## STANDARDS

**LEVEL 1:** 2 sets of 15
**LEVEL 2:** 2 sets of 25
**LEVEL 3:** 3 sets of 35

Do 2-3 sets of as many as you can.

Once you can meet or exceed Level 3 with **GOOD FORM,** you are ready to move on to a harder variation.

# BEHIND THE EXERCISE

The ability to get off the ground is a fundamental to survival and mobility!

We can start building this ability by assisting with our arms - even if this means assisting heavily at first!

For some - this exercise will seem daunting. To others, it may seem incredibly easy.

Either way, try the Standards below and see if you can hit them. If you hit Level 3 easily, feel free to move on!

If not, then congratulations - you're strengthening one of the most fundamental human movements!

# FORM CUES

Your legs should be approximately shoulder width apart.

Your feet should point forward or slightly out. Don't point them excessively out.

Find a base from which you can firmly push. If you use a chair or low table, make sure it will not collapse on you and hurt you.

Tighten your core and abs during the movement. This applies to all squats. You want to feel your body "hinge" at the hips - like a jackknife opening! This is the namesake of the exercise and will involve solid upper and lower body engagement.

# PROGRESSION & REGRESSION

**To make this exercise harder:** Doing this with a slightly higher platform may make assistance more difficult. This will smoothly lead us into the next step!

**To make this exercise easier:** This exercise is easier if you do not squat down as deeply, or if you increase assistance from your arms in this range. Over time, increase squat depth and reduce arm assistance. Alternatively, you can squat into a very low chair or stool. This "resting spot" will make the bottom portion easier and track your progress.

# ASSISTED SQUATS

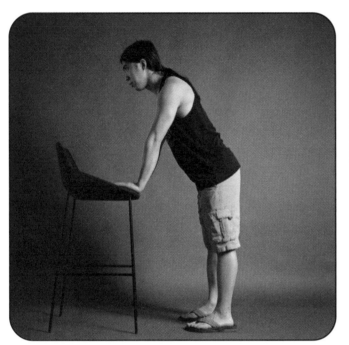

**ASCEND**

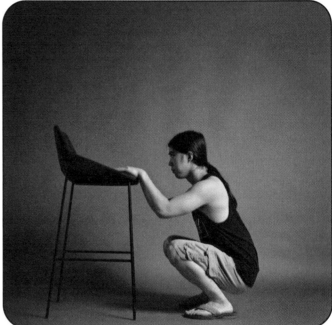

**DESCEND**

## TUTORIAL

1.  Stand in front of a stable platform around hip height.

2.  Maintaining straight legs, bend at the hips until your palms are on the platform. Your arms should be relatively straight, as should your waist.

3.  Squat down slowly, with a slightly forward lean so you may assist with your arms, until your hamstrings are pressed against your calves. You should not be able to squat any further.

4.  Pause for 1 Second.

5.  Slowly come back up.

6.  Pause for 1 Second.

7.  Repeat 3-6.

# STANDARDS

**LEVEL 1:** 2 sets of 10
**LEVEL 2:** 2 sets of 20
**LEVEL 3:** 3 sets of 30

Do 2–3 sets of as many as you can.

Once you can meet or exceed Level 3 with **GOOD FORM,** you are ready to move on to a harder variation.

# BEHIND THE EXERCISE

This exercise continues where Jackknife Squats left off.

The key difference is the increased height of the assisting platform. Users should feel like they're "pulling" themselves up at the bottom, rather than pressing!

# FORM CUES

This is a good place to start using Gymnastic Rings, if you happen to have them. You can adjust them to your ideal height. Alternatively, you can use a rope or sturdy railing.

Your legs should be approximately shoulder width apart.

Your feet should point forward or slightly out. Don't point them excessively out.

# PROGRESSION & REGRESSION

**To make this exercise harder:** Assisting less with your arms will make this exercise harder. As you get stronger, try not assisting at all on the way up after your thighs are parallel. This is basically the concentric portion of Half Squats!

**To make this exercise easier:** Assisting more with your arms will make this exercise easier.

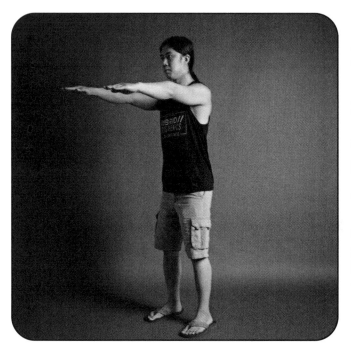

**ASCEND**

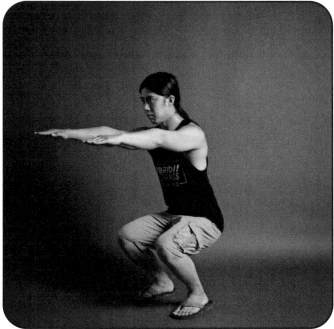

**DESCEND**

# TUTORIAL

1. Stand in a safe area with your feet shoulder width apart.

2. Place your arms wherever they feel comfortable. Some extend their arms straight in front of them, and others place them across their chest.

3. Squat down slowly until your thighs are parallel with the ground.

4. Pause for 1 Second.

5. Slowly come back up.

6. Pause for 1 Second.

7. Repeat 3-6.

## STANDARDS

**LEVEL 1:** 2 sets of 10
**LEVEL 2:** 2 sets of 20
**LEVEL 3:** 3 sets of 50

Do 2-3 sets of as many as you can.

Once you can meet or exceed Level 3 with **GOOD FORM,** you are ready to move on to a harder variation.

## BEHIND THE EXERCISE

This is the first step where we are squatting our entire bodyweight without assistance!

However, we are stronger in the upper half of our range, and this exercise takes advantage of that.

Our balance and core will have to work harder as a result - preparing us for the harder steps!

## FORM CUES

Because this is the first Squat variation where we do not train a full range of motion, always follow this exercise with a few sets of Assisted Squats or Jackknife Squats to maintain strength in this range!

Some people bend heavily at the hips to make this exercise easier. Don't make this mistake! Allow a slight forward lean, but squat with your entire lower body.

## PROGRESSION & REGRESSION

**To make this exercise harder:** Squatting below parallel will make this exercise harder and lead you smoothly into the next step!

**To make this exercise easier:** Reducing the squat depth will make this exercise easier. Add an inch or two of depth whenever you feel ready, and you will eventually be able to squat to parallel. Alternatively, placing a chair underneath you so you may rest in the bottom position can make this exercise easier. However, don't rely on this too much. You want to eventually be able to do this without the chair.

# FULL SQUATS

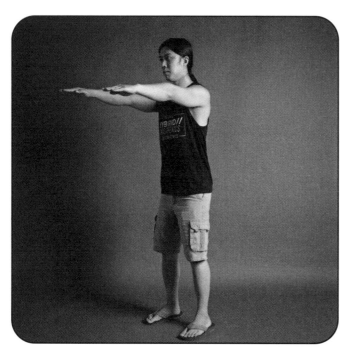

**ASCEND**

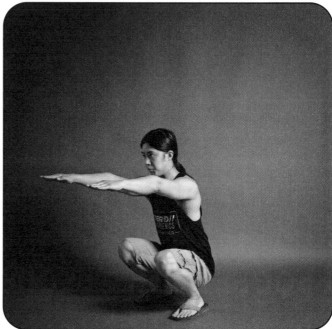

**DESCEND**

## TUTORIAL

1.  Stand in a safe area with your feet shoulder width apart.

2.  Place your arms wherever they feel comfortable. Some extend their arms straight in front of them, and others place them across their chest.

3.  Squat down slowly until your hamstrings are pressed against your calves and you are unable to descend any further.

4.  Pause for 1 Second.

5.  Slowly come back up.

6.  Pause for 1 Second.

7.  Repeat 3-6.

## STANDARDS

**LEVEL 1:** 2 sets of 10
**LEVEL 2:** 2 sets of 20
**LEVEL 3:** 3 sets of 30

Do 2-3 sets of as many as you can.

Once you can meet or exceed Level 3 with **GOOD FORM,** you are ready to move on to a harder variation.

# BEHIND THE EXERCISE

This is another calisthenics staple! Being able to get up off the floor without the assistance from your arms is important to survival and overall mobility!

Not only this, but the full range of motion will keep the tendons and ligaments of your ankles, hips, and knees strong and healthy for years to come.

Even after you get "too strong" for these, practice them infrequently so you don't lose the strength for this movement. Your body will thank you for it.

Congratulations on achieving this bodyweight standard!

# FORM CUES

You may be tempted to "bounce" out of the difficult bottom range. While you might be able to do more reps this way, this will only make you weaker. Aim to control every inch of the movement.

Try to keep your back neutral throughout the exercise. This means don't arch or round your back. This may take some work if you're not used to it, but you should make progress over time. Your lower back may round at the very bottom. This is usually fine.

# PROGRESSION & REGRESSION

**To make this exercise harder:** Squatting with your feet less than shoulder width apart will make this exercise harder and lead you smoothly into the next step!

**To make this exercise easier:** Assisting yourself out of the bottom position - the hardest part - will make this exercise easier.

# NARROW SQUATS

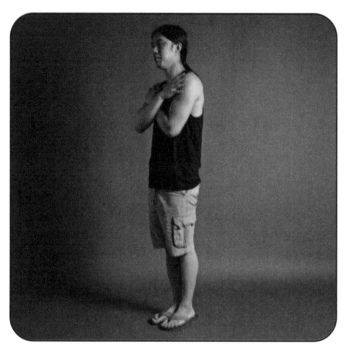

**ASCEND**

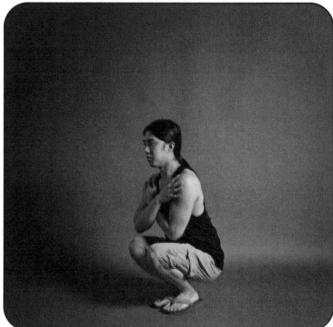

**DESCEND**

## TUTORIAL

1.  Stand in a safe area with your legs straight and heels touching.

2.  Place your arms wherever they feel comfortable. Some extend their arms straight in front of them, and others place them across their chest.

3.  Squat down slowly until your hamstrings are pressed against your calves and you are unable to descend any further.

4.  Pause for 1 Second.

5.  Slowly come back up.

6.  Pause for 1 Second.

7.  Repeat 3-6.

## STANDARDS

**LEVEL 1:** 2 sets of 10
**LEVEL 2:** 2 sets of 20
**LEVEL 3:** 3 sets of 30

Do 2-3 sets of as many as you can.

Once you can meet or exceed Level 3 with **GOOD FORM,** you are ready to move on to a harder variation.

## BEHIND THE EXERCISE

While not a very well known exercise, Narrow Squats amplify the benefits of Deep Squats by increasing the work on our quadriceps and joints!

This helps prepare our legs for the rigors of one-leg squatting!

## FORM CUES

This exercise is done with the heels touching. The feet can be pointed forward or slightly out.

If you lose balance during this exercise, do this near a wall so you can use it balance when needed. Over time, learn this squat without the wall.

Tighten your core and abs during the movement. You want to feel your body "hinge" at the hips.

As we are building up progressively, it is okay for your knees to go over your toes. Doing this with an exercise we can competently handle will strengthen our joints in tandem with our muscles.

## PROGRESSION & REGRESSION

**To make this exercise harder:** This is our last step in the Squat series before we explore one-leg squatting. Really spend some time mastering your form on this exercise to make it harder. When you're ready, you can start moving one leg further away, as shown the next step!

**To make this exercise easier:** Standing with your feet further apart will make this exercise easier. Bring your heels an inch or two closer whenever you feel ready. Aim to learn this with your heels touching! If your femurs are particularly long, it may help you to hold some light weights in front of you with your arm to counterbalance.

# SIDE STAGGERED SQUATS

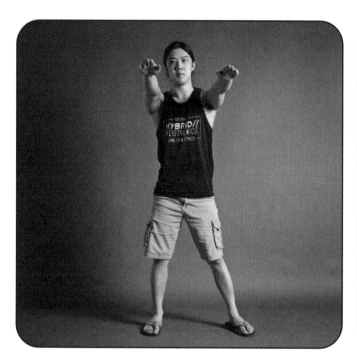

**ASCEND**

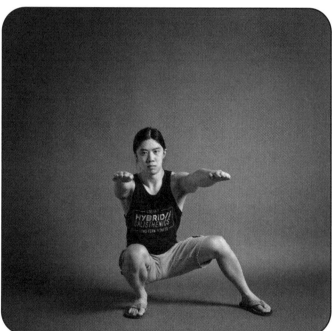

**DESCEND**

## TUTORIAL

1. Stand in a safe area with your legs straight and feet twice shoulder width apart.

2. Place your arms wherever they feel comfortable. Some extend their arms straight in front of them, and others place them across their chest.

3. Squat down slowly towards one side until your hamstrings are pressed against your calves and you are unable to descend any further.

4. Pause for 1 Second.

5. Slowly come back up.

6. Pause for 1 Second.

7. Repeat 3-6.

## STANDARDS

**LEVEL 1:** 2 Sets of 10 (Both Sides)
**LEVEL 2:** 2 Sets of 15 (Both Sides)
**LEVEL 3:** 2 Sets of 20 (Both Sides)

Do 2-3 sets of as many as you can.

Once you can meet or exceed Level 3 with **GOOD FORM,** you are ready to move on to a harder variation.

## BEHIND THE EXERCISE

Having developed a foundation of strength through Deep Squats and Narrow Squats, it's time to explore progressions that emphasize one leg more than the other!

These are essentially squats done with a wide stance and descending at an angle. If you're familiar with Archer Pushups and Archer Pullups, you can think of these as "Archer Squats."

Squatting to the side like this seems to be easier than having one leg in front of the other, so we explore these first!

## FORM CUES

Work one side at a time during a set. This trains your working muscles to operate under constant tension.

The wider your foot positioning, the harder this exercise will be. Start with approximately twice shoulder width if you can!

Move your arms however you wish to balance this exercise. It does not matter much.

## PROGRESSION & REGRESSION

**To make this exercise harder:** A wider stance will make this exercise harder. Alternatively, you can begin to experiment keeping your movement more "vertical" similar to how Sliding One-Arm Pushups are done. This will challenge your strength and balance more!

**To make this exercise easier:** Having your feet closer together will make this exercise easier.

# FRONT STAGGERED SQUATS

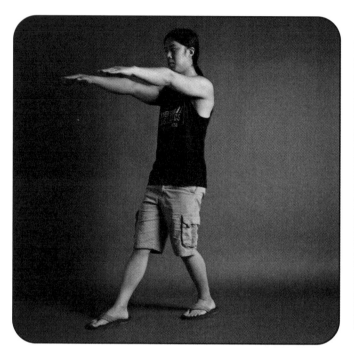

**ASCEND**

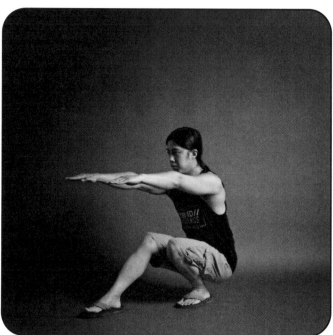

**DESCEND**

## TUTORIAL

1. Stand in a safe area with one foot in front of the other. Your legs should be relatively straight.
2. Squat down slowly on your back leg until your hamstrings are pressed against your calves and you are unable to descend any further.
3. Pause for 1 Second.
4. Slowly come back up.
5. Pause for 1 Second.
6. Repeat 3-6.

## STANDARDS

**LEVEL 1:** 2 Sets of 7 (Both Sides)
**LEVEL 2:** 2 Sets of 12 (Both Sides)
**LEVEL 3:** 2 Sets of 15 (Both Sides)

Do 2-3 sets of as many as you can.

Once you can meet or exceed Level 3 with **GOOD FORM,** you are ready to move on to a harder variation.

## BEHIND THE EXERCISE

Similar to Side-Staggered Squats, here we continue to progress towards one-leg squatting.

The assisting leg in front of us better transfers to "full" One-Leg Squats and increases the strength, balance, and mobility requirements.

## FORM CUES

The further your assisting foot, the harder the exercise. Work up to having your assisting foot 2 feet away from your working foot.

Similarly, having your feet shoulder width apart will help your balance. Over time, move your assisting foot directly in front of your working one. This will better simulate the balance necessary for One-Leg Squats.

Work one side at a time during a set. This trains your working muscles to operate under constant tension.

Move your arms however you wish to balance this exercise. It does not matter much.

## PROGRESSION & REGRESSION

**To make this exercise harder:** Having your assisting foot further away will make this exercise harder. Alternatively, you can raise your heels on the assisting foot - assisting only with your toes.

**To make this exercise easier:** Having your feet closer together will make this exercise easier.

# ASSISTED ONE LEG SQUATS

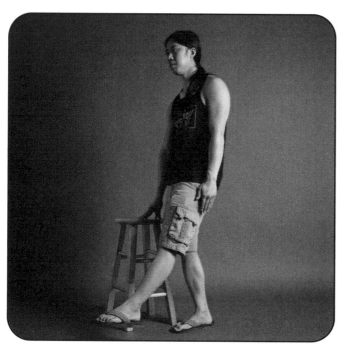

**ASCEND**

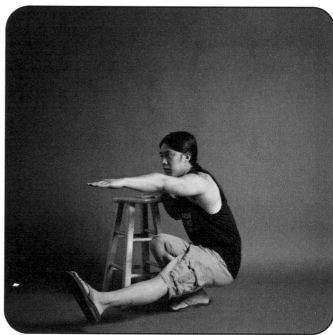

**DESCEND**

## TUTORIAL

1. Stand in a safe area in front of Gymnastic Rings or a stable assisting platform.

2. Grab the assisting platform with your hands and raise one leg off the ground. Both legs should be straight.

3. Squat down slowly on your back leg until your hamstrings are pressed against your calves and you are unable to descend any further.

4. Pause for 1 Second.

5. Slowly come back up.

6. Pause for 1 Second.

7. Repeat 3-6.

## STANDARDS

**LEVEL 1:** 2 Sets of 5 (Both Sides)
**LEVEL 2:** 2 Sets of 9 (Both Sides)
**LEVEL 3:** 2 Sets of 12 (Both Sides)

Do 2-3 sets of as many as you can.

Once you can meet or exceed Level 3 with **GOOD FORM,** you are ready to move on to a harder variation.

## BEHIND THE EXERCISE

This is a valuable step where the user has to balance and squat on one-leg.

Hold your horses, Nelly. Slow and steady wins the race, so we're going to assist yourselves through the movement!

In this manner, we will get a taste of the raw strength and balance necessary for One-Leg Squats while allowing our weak links to be identified and developed through assistance!

Finding something around waist height to assist yourself is a good start.

Some may also like using a pole or tree to assist themselves. This is usually a little more difficult.

## FORM CUES

The standard for this exercise is assisting yourself with something around waist height. This can be Gymnastic Rings or a stable railing or table. Assist yourself with whatever you can to get started!

One-Leg Squats look better with your assisting leg straight and parallel with the ground at the bottom of the movement. While this is a good workout for your hip flexors, it's not necessary to get started. Try to keep it off to the ground, and work on getting your leg straighter and more mobile over time.

Work one side at a time during a set. This trains your working muscles to operate under constant tension.

## PROGRESSION & REGRESSION

**To make this exercise harder:** Assisting less with your arms will make this exercise harder. You can try assisting with one arm at a time to better gauge this.

**To make this exercise easier:** Assisting more with your arms will make this exercise easier. Having the assisting platform closer will make this easier.

# ONE LEG CHAIR SQUATS

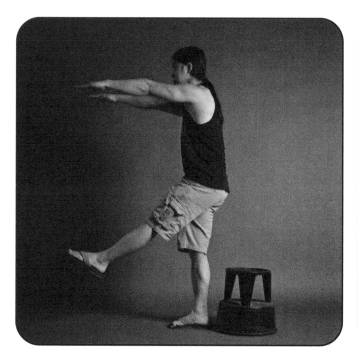

**ASCEND**

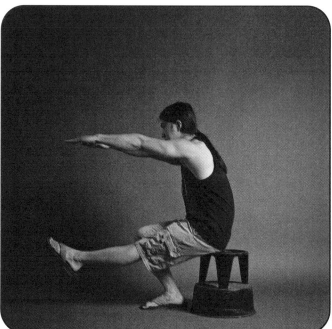

**DESCEND**

## TUTORIAL

1. Stand in a safe area with a safe, stable chair behind you. The chair should be around knee height.

2. Raise one leg off the ground. Both legs should be straight. Use your arms to balance however you choose.

3. Squat down slowly on one leg until your butt gently touches the chair.

4. Pause for 1 Second.

5. Slowly come back up.

6. Pause for 1 Second.

7. Repeat 3-6.

## STANDARDS

**LEVEL 1:** 2 Sets of 5 (Both Sides)
**LEVEL 2:** 2 Sets of 9 (Both Sides)
**LEVEL 3:** 2 Sets of 12 (Both Sides)

Do 2-3 sets of as many as you can.

Once you can meet or exceed Level 3 with **GOOD FORM,** you are ready to move on to a harder variation.

## BEHIND THE EXERCISE

Now that we've built the ability to assist ourselves through a one-leg squat, it's time to experiment with unassisted squatting!

We're stronger in the upper half of our range of motion, so we start here! The strength we build here will transfer to our weaker range.

Because the brief pause in the lowest part of this squat is hard for some, we use a chair to make this easier. It's basically sitting down and standing up on one leg!

## FORM CUES

The standard for this exercise is squatting from a chair around knee height. If this is too difficult and you find yourself falling the last few inches, then experiment with a higher chair. As you get stronger, lower the chair!

You'll know you're making progress with this exercise when you can gently touch the chair with your butt, instead of sitting all the way down!

## PROGRESSION & REGRESSION

**To make this exercise harder:** Using a lower chair or removing the chair entirely will make this exercise harder! If you can remove the chair and gradually squat lower and lower as the weeks go by, this will lead you smoothly to the next step!

**To make this exercise easier:** Using a higher chair and using it to take more of your weight will make this exercise easier.

# ONE LEG SQUATS

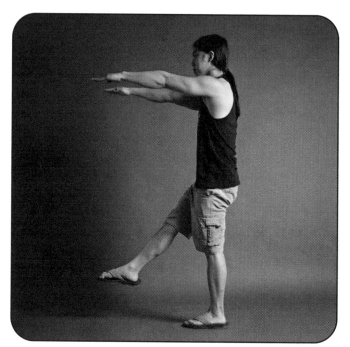

**ASCEND**

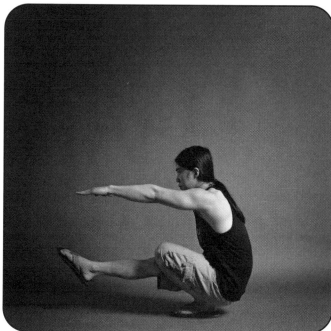

**DESCEND**

## TUTORIAL

1. Stand in a safe area.
2. Raise one leg off the ground. Both legs should be straight. Use your arms to balance however you choose.
3. Squat down slowly on one leg until your hamstrings are pressed firmly against your calves.
4. Pause for 1 Second.
5. Slowly come back up.
6. Pause for 1 Second.
7. Repeat 3-6.

## STANDARDS

**LEVEL 1:** 2 Sets of 5 (Both Sides)
**LEVEL 2:** 2 Sets of 9 (Both Sides)
**LEVEL 3:** 2 Sets of 12 (Both Sides)

Do 2-3 sets of as many as you can.

Once you can meet or exceed Level 3 with **GOOD FORM,** you are ready to move on to a harder variation.

# BEHIND THE EXERCISE

Squatting on one leg is arguably more functional than bilateral squats. If you consider most of human lower body movement - walking, running, climbing stairs - almost all of this involves one leg to work harder than the other!

One-Leg Squats take this fundamental human movement and scale it through our entire range of motion.

Not only will this build strength, muscle, and mobility through our ENTIRE lower body, it'll also keep our joints healthy, strong, and moving for years to come.

As with all calisthenics moves, build up to this progressively. If your joints hurt from doing this movement, experiment with some easier variations instead.

Congratulations on reaching this step!

# FORM CUES

This exercise is particularly difficult in the bottom range. As a result, you may be tempted to "bounce" out of the bottom. To build strength in this weak point, resist this urge and maintain a brief pause at the bottom.

As you do more reps, it may be hard to maintain your balance sometimes. Do these by a wall and lightly touch it to maintain your balance when necessary.

Try to resist your knees "collapsing inward." Our knees are hinge joints and don't resist sideways pressure well. A good rule of thumb is to have your knee go over your second toe (next to your big toe).

One-Leg Squats look better with your assisting leg straight and parallel with the ground at the bottom of the movement. While this is a good workout for your hip flexors, it's not necessary to get started. Try to keep it off to the ground, and work on getting your leg straighter and more mobile over time.

# PROGRESSION & REGRESSION

**To make this exercise harder:** Build up plenty of repetitions (20+) with this exercise before trying to make it more difficult. Then you can explore variety in your training rather than scaling this particular exercise. Try Reverse Nordic Curls, Nordic Curls, Sissy Squats, and more! If you love One-Leg Squats and just want to scale the difficulty, you can try holding a dumbbell while doing them. I personally find this a bit boring, though.

**To make this exercise easier:** Not squatting all the way down will make this exercise easier. As you get stronger, you can go lower! It may help you to use your hands pressing on the ground to assist yourself out of the bottom portion. This will build unassisted strength through most of your range while still training the bottom!

# CLOSING THOUGHTS

Congratulations! If you have made it this far, then you have completed the entirety of the Squat series. Give yourself a pat on the back for achieving mastery of such a valuable movement pattern.

We squat all the time! We squat to pick up a child or a beloved pet. We squat to get in and out of chairs. We use our lower bodies to walk, run, and more! Mastering squats will prepare you for important activities of daily living, whether you are 20 or 120 years old!

Perhaps you want to explore more variations on a squat. Here are a few exercises that might give you an idea of where you want to go next:

**Hill Sprints** – Running fast up a hill and timing yourself trains cardio AND explosive legs!

**Sumo Squats** – You mastered Narrow Squats, so you'll want to master wide-stance squats, too! With a wide base of support and toes turned out, you'll be working the muscles of the inner thigh as well as the gluteus medius, a smaller but very important muscle in the glute complex.

One thing to keep in mind is the alignment of your knees. Your knees should track with your toes, and because your toes are turned out, your knees should turn out as well. This will put the stabilizing muscles of your hip to work. This is why this exercise is so great for improving lower body stability and balance.

**Cossack Squats** – These might remind you of the Side Staggered Squats. The difference here is in the stance. You'll be standing much wider and keeping your "kickstand" leg straight. You can imagine squatting down to sit on your heel. There is a significant balance component, and you'll feel it immediately.

Because this is a lateral movement, you are recruiting different muscles that you would in a traditional squat. It's a great exercise for improving your lower body stability and the range of motion in your hips, knees, and ankles.

**Lunges** – Yes, lunges! The single-leg exercise that strengthens the glutes, quads, hamstrings and calves. It's actually one of the five fundamental movement patterns!

The split stance of a lunge challenges your core and hips as you work to maintain balanced form. There are many variations on a lunge, from the classic forward lunge to the deep lunge. Explore your options and see where you might incorporate them into your routine.

---

Having a strong and stable lower body is endlessly useful. Whether you're dancing the night away or leaping over hurdles to escape from zombies, you can thank your past self for taking the time to master the squat.

**Where do I start?**

Start with a variation that you can do competently with good form for at least a few repetitions. When in doubt, start with Jackknife Squats!

**I'm having trouble keeping my heels on the ground during my squats. How can I fix this?**

You might need to work on your ankle flexibility! You can do this by going back to the first variations and focusing solely on your range of motion. Try moving slowly and pausing at the bottom to train in proper heel placement.

You can also do calf stretches in between your sets to improve your flexibility.

**I have met the standard for one variation, but the next exercise feels too hard. What should I do?**

Each exercise has a Progression and a Regression. You can use these to your advantage!

For example, let's say you are stuck somewhere between two exercises. If your Jackknife Squats are too easy, the Progression will challenge your body in preparation for the next exercise (using a higher platform).

Alternatively, if the Assisted Squats are too challenging, the Regression will allow you to build into them more slowly (using your arms for more assistance).

You can think of these as transition exercises!

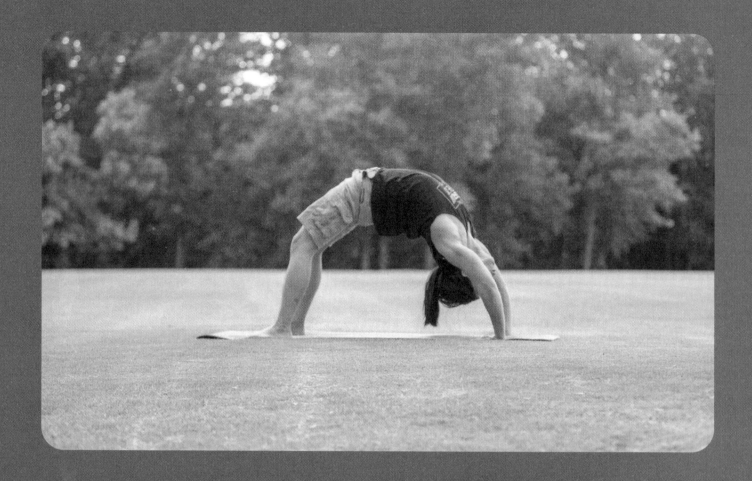

# BRIDGES

Bridging is excellent for the health of your spine – IF you take the time to really master each step. To execute an impressive back bend safely, training takes both patience and care.

In today's modern age, we spend a lot of time in flexion. That is, we are often in a rounded forward position for long periods of time. Think of a day at the office or at school. Think of what your posture looks like at your computer, looking at your phone, or even reading a book – we often tend to round our backs during these activities.

Bridging will put your spine in extension. This is a good thing, because we want our bodies to be in balance! Too much time in flexion can cause issues in the future, so it's a good idea to counter that by learning how to (safely) do the opposite! Take each variation to heart as you strengthen the muscles of your back and improve mobility in your shoulders, hips, and spine. This trains your posterior chain!

# GENERAL BRIDGE CUES

Some are repeated on certain exercises as a reminder.

Try to avoid sagging at the hips. If this is difficult, moving your feet closer or pressing more with your arms sometimes helps.

Slow and steady wins the race on this exercise. Don't just speed through these. Find a controlled, rhythmic pace to really feel this movement. 2 Seconds Down, 1 Second Pause, 2 Seconds Up. Repeat.

Keep your feet relatively straight. They should point forward.

Bridges are an excellent exercise, but slightly riskier for those who aren't prepared. I do not advise rushing through these exercises. If at all concerned, feel free to skip these. As mentioned in the beginning of this book, consult a doctor before starting a new exercise plan.

# BRIDGE PROGRESSIONS

We'll begin by strengthening the posterior chain and introducing the beginnings of the bridging movement pattern. Go slowly and be thorough – the first three movements are unique and important to master.

Once we have mastered the Wall Bridge, we'll challenge ourselves by lowering the base. Good form is important, but how we get into position is even more important. Safety is the name of the game, and being consistent and methodical in your approach will reduce your risk for injury. After you have mastered the Wheel Bridge, you're on your way to the "Look mom, no hands!" version of this exercise. Don't rush the process. Control will be key in mastering this movement.

Let's bridge the gap!

1. Glute Bridges
2. Straight Bridges
3. Wall Bridges
4. Incline Bridges
5. Head Bridges
6. Full Bridges
7. Wheel Bridges
8. Tap Bridges
9. Wall Walking Bridges
10. Stand to Stand Bridges

# GLUTE BRIDGES

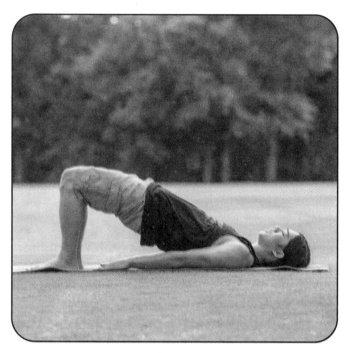

**ASCEND**

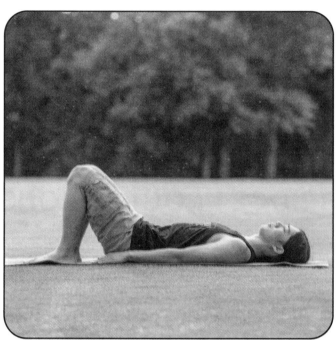

**DESCEND**

## TUTORIAL

1. Lie on your back with your knees bent. Your legs should be shoulder width apart.

2. Contract your glutes while maintaining a neutral back. This should thrust your hips upward.

3. Continue this movement until your thighs, trunk, and torso are in a straight line.

4. Pause for 1 Second.

5. Slowly come back down.

6. Pause for 1 Second.

7. Repeat 2-6.

# STANDARDS

**LEVEL 1:** 2 Sets of 15
**LEVEL 2:** 2 Sets of 30
**LEVEL 3:** 2 Sets of 50

Do 2-3 sets of as many as you can.

Once you can meet or exceed Level 3 with **GOOD FORM,** you are ready to move on to a harder variation.

# BEHIND THE EXERCISE

A gentle exercise to introduce ourselves to bridging!

Our back muscles are mostly working isometrically, so this gives most of the movement work to our glutes. Our back still gets a good workout.

This is a great introductory exercise that prepares us for more difficult bridging.

# FORM CUES

Your foot placement affects difficulty. Try to keep your shins perpendicular to the ground and/or have your heels a few inches from your butt.

Try to avoid sagging at the hips. If this is difficult, moving your feet closer or pressing more with your arms sometimes helps.

Have your legs around shoulder width apart.

Try to keep your back neutral throughout the exercise.

Tighten your core and abs during the movement. You want to feel your body "hinge" at the hips. This is similar to the movement of Jackknife Squats and Jackknife Pullups!

# PROGRESSION & REGRESSION

**To make this exercise harder:** Doing this exercise with your heels further away from your butt can make it more difficult.

**To make this exercise easier:** This exercise is easier if held for time instead of doing reps. If you have difficulty doing Level 1 with good form, try getting into the top position and holding this for a few minutes at a time. This should improve your ability to form a straight line from your shoulders to your knees.

# STRAIGHT BRIDGES

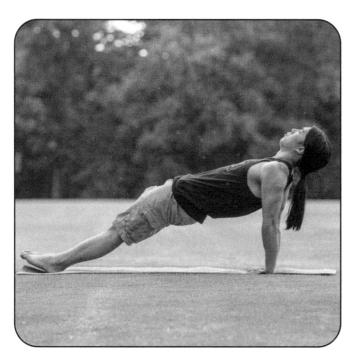

**ASCEND**

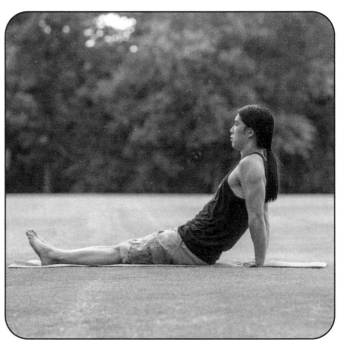

**DESCEND**

## TUTORIAL

1. Sit on the floor with your legs in front of you. Your palms should be by your hips. Your body should form an angle slightly wider than a right angle.

2. Push through your arms and contract your glutes to begin the movement. Keep your arms and legs straight and bring your shoulders back.

3. Continue this movement until your body is in a straight line supported by your heels and palms.

4. Pause for 1 Second.

5. Slowly come back down.

6. Pause for 1 Second.

7. Repeat 2-6.

## STANDARDS

**LEVEL 1:** 2 Sets of 15
**LEVEL 2:** 2 Sets of 25
**LEVEL 3:** 3 Sets of 30

Do 2-3 sets of as many as you can.

Once you can meet or exceed Level 3 with **GOOD FORM,** you are ready to move on to a harder variation.

# BEHIND THE EXERCISE

This brings the entire body into action!

This exercise works the entire posterior chain and brings our arms in to the ring.

However, because we are not bending backwards yet, the mobility and strength requirements are not as high.

This exercise is a great way to prepare our bridging muscles for the more advanced variations.

You could even say it's a "bridge" to other exercises. *Badumtss.*

# FORM CUES

Ideal form in this exercise starts from your body at slightly wider than a right angle and transitions into a straight line. This will involve your shoulder blades retracting, which may help you with your overall posture.

Try to avoid sagging at the hips. If this is difficult, try bending your knees a bit.

Have your legs together.

Your feet should point forward or slightly out. Point your toes forward.

Try to keep your back neutral throughout the exercise.

Tighten your core and abs during the movement. You want to feel your body "hinge" at the hips. This is similar to the movement of Jackknife Squats and Jackknife Pullups!

# PROGRESSION & REGRESSION

**To make this exercise harder:** Raising your heels will make this exercise harder. A chair, ottoman, or stool works well. However, this will make it harder to form a straight line at the top of the movement.

**To make this exercise easier:** Bending your knees slightly will make this exercise easier.

# WALL BRIDGES

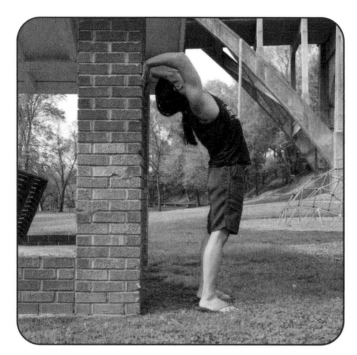

**ASCEND**

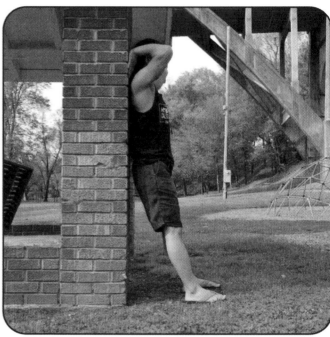

**DESCEND**

## TUTORIAL

1. Stand 12" away from a wall. Your arms should be by your side and your legs shoulder width apart.

2. Bring your arms back until your palms touch the wall. Your fingers should be pointed down.

3. Lean backwards, trying to move one spinal vertebra at a time, until your head gently touches the wall.

4. Pause for 1 Second.

5. Slowly reverse the movement.

6. Pause for 1 Second.

7. Repeat 3-6.

## STANDARDS

**LEVEL 1:** 2 Sets of 15
**LEVEL 2:** 2 Sets of 25
**LEVEL 3:** 3 Sets of 30

Do 2-3 sets of as many as you can.

Once you can meet or exceed Level 3 with **GOOD FORM**, you are ready to move on to a harder variation.

# BEHIND THE EXERCISE

Now that we've acclimated our body to use our posterior chain in synergy, it's time work on the next step - bending backwards!

It's much easier to build this mobility against a wall first.

Because this movement is unusual for many individuals, it may take you a while to get comfortable or mobile enough. This is fine. The other exercises in the routine will condition your body while you make progress on this exercise. It may take a few weeks to get comfortable with this - particularly if you're older, new to exercise, or both

# FORM CUES

Breathe normally throughout this exercise. This is very important. The new positioning in our body can make our blood rush to and from our head. If we hold our breath and suddenly release it, this may result in severe dizziness.

If you feel dizzy, stop immediately and take a break. Walk around the room while breathing normally before returning to your exercise set. This applies to all bridges.

Try to externally rotate your shoulders during this exercise. This meaning rotating your upper arms away from your body. It may help you to envision trying to bring your elbows together. This applies to many bridges.

Try to arch your back evenly. Don't hinge at one point while keeping the rest straight. Imagine your back being as curved as the letter U.

# PROGRESSION & REGRESSION

**To make this exercise harder:** Standing further away from the wall will make this exercise harder.

**To make this exercise easier:** Standing closer to the wall or not leaning back all the way will make this exercise easier. Build range of motion over time.

# INCLINE BRIDGES

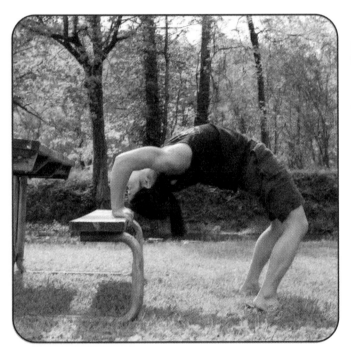

**ASCEND**

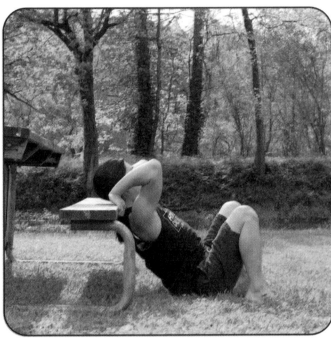

**DESCEND**

## TUTORIAL

1. Sit in front of a platform around thigh height. A bench is a good standard. Your arms should be by your side and your legs shoulder width apart.

2. Lean back until your head and palms touch the object. Lift your hips until your body is support by your head, palms, and feet.

3. Lean backwards, trying to move one spinal vertebra at a time, until your body is arched and your head is clear of the platform.

4. Pause for 1 Second.

5. Slowly reverse the movement.

6. Pause for 1 Second.

7. Repeat 3-6.

## STANDARDS

**LEVEL 1:** 2 Sets of 10
**LEVEL 2:** 2 Sets of 20
**LEVEL 3:** 3 Sets of 25

Do 2–3 sets of as many as you can.

Once you can meet or exceed Level 3 with **GOOD FORM,** you are ready to move on to a harder variation.

## BEHIND THE EXERCISE

Lowering our upper body makes the bridge more difficult.

However, because of the angle, not much movement is possible. Some muscles may feel like they're not moving much at all.

This is still building strength and will help us transition to the next steps!

## FORM CUES

Your wrist positioning is key on this exercise. Don't have your wrists so far back that they have to contort to support your body. If you're using a bench, place them on the edge.

Use a stable platform. Make sure it does not wiggle around or move. Anything glass or fragile is out of the question.

Using a "squishy" surface like a bed might make this exercise harder on your wrists. A stable bench is a good standard for this exercise.

If you feel dizzy, take a break. Breathe normally throughout the exercise.

Try to arch your back evenly. Don't hinge at one point while keeping the rest straight. Imagine your back being as curved as the letter U. This applies to all bridges with an arched back.

## PROGRESSION & REGRESSION

**To make this exercise harder:** Using a lower platform will make this exercise harder.

**To make this exercise easier:** Using a higher platform will make this exercise easier. Adjust your wrists as necessary. They should not hurt during this exercise.

# HEAD BRIDGES

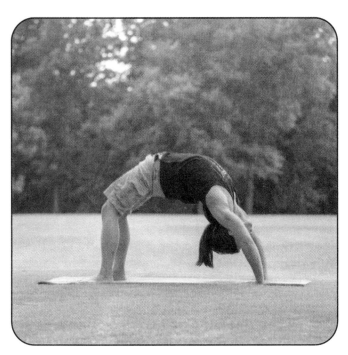

**ASCEND**

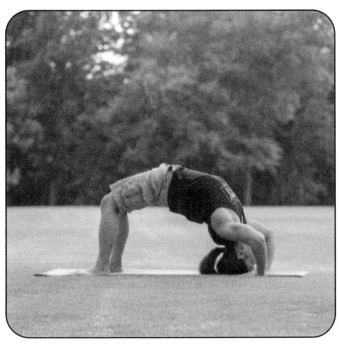

**DESCEND**

## TUTORIAL

1.  Sit on a platform around knee height. Your legs should be around shoulder width.

2.  Lean back until your head and palms touch the floor. Use the platform to support your lower body as you arch back.

3.  Lean backwards, pushing through your palms and feet until your head and back are clear of the floor. You should be in a Full Bridge position - supported only be your palms and feet!

4.  Pause for 5 Seconds. Breathing evenly and feeling your muscles stretch.

5.  Slowly reverse the movement.

6.  Pause for 1 Second.

7.  Repeat 3-6.

## STANDARDS

**LEVEL 1:** 2 Sets of 5
**LEVEL 2:** 2 Sets of 10
**LEVEL 3:** 2 Sets of 25

Do 2-3 sets of as many as you can.

Once you can meet or exceed Level 3 with **GOOD FORM,** you are ready to move on to a harder variation.

# BEHIND THE EXERCISE

How we get into position here is really more important than the motion itself.

By using a raised object to assist us into a bridge position, we're able to explore this range of motion.

This is easier than raising into a Bridge position from the floor.

Use only safe, stable objects. This exercise should NOT hurt. If it does hurt your back, return to an easier variation for now.

# FORM CUES

It's important to find the right platform for this exercise. Make sure it is safe, secure, and stable. You do not want to fall on the platform. However, if you do, make sure it can support your weight. A cushioned stool may work well.

Try to keep your bridge "even." Don't lean too far towards your feet or your palms. Try to keep it balanced. If your wrists hurt, you may need to move towards your palms a bit.

Full-body activation really comes into play here. Try to imagine each vertebra of your body moving back at a time. This applies to many bridges.

# PROGRESSION & REGRESSION

**To make this exercise harder:** Using a lower platform will make this exercise harder, as you have to move through a greater range of motion.

**To make this exercise easier:** Using a higher platform will make this exercise easier. Adjust your wrists as necessary. They should not hurt during this exercise.

# FULL BRIDGES

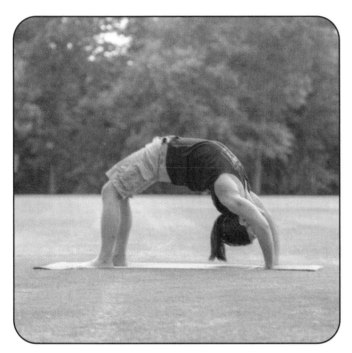

**ASCEND**

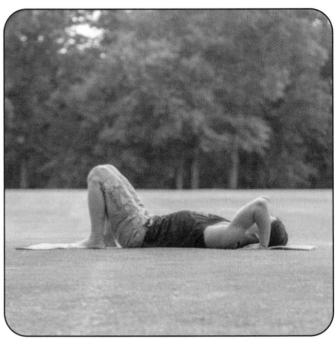

**DESCEND**

## TUTORIAL

1. Lie on your back with your knees bent. Your heels should be a few inches away from your butt.

2. Reach back until your palms touch the floor. Your hands should be next to your head with your fingers pointing towards your feet.

3. Push through your palms and feet while arching your back until your arms and legs are as straight as you can make them. You should be in a Full Bridge position - supported only by your palms and feet!

4. Pause for 5 Seconds. Breathing evenly and feeling your muscles stretch.

5. Slowly reverse the movement.

6. Pause for 5 Seconds.

7. Repeat 3-6.

# STANDARDS

**LEVEL 1:** 2 Sets of 5
**LEVEL 2:** 2 Sets of 10
**LEVEL 3:** 2 Sets of 15

Do 2-3 sets of as many as you can.

Once you can meet or exceed Level 3 with **GOOD FORM,** you are ready to move on to a harder variation.

# BEHIND THE EXERCISE

This is the full bridge exercise often done by calisthenics athletes!

While there are more advanced versions, this is an excellent mobility standard to accomplish for most people. Congratulations!

The difference between this stage and Head Bridges is simply range of motion. By pushing off from the ground, we are moving more and expending more energy.

As you'll see from the next stage, there is a significant difference between an "acceptable" Bridge and a "good" Bridge.

Take your time refining this exercise and the next to improve yours!

# FORM CUES

The difficulty of this exercise is affected by the distance between your hands and feet. Don't start with them too close. Experiment with the distance.

Try to straighten your arms.

Try to straighten your legs.

Try to retract your scapula and bring your shoulders back.

Try to keep your bridge "even." Don't lean too far towards your feet or your palms. Try to keep it balanced. If your wrists hurt, you may need to move towards your palms a bit.

Full-body activation really comes into play here. Try to imagine each vertebra of your body moving back at a time.

# PROGRESSION & REGRESSION

**To make this exercise harder:** Doing this exercise with perfect form will make this exercise harder! Aim for straighter legs and arms. Breathe normally. Maintain a smooth curve in the back. Be an upside down U rather than an upside down V.

**To make this exercise easier:** Moving your hands and feet slightly further apart will make this exercise easier. You may need to lean towards your hands more so that your wrists don't have to bend excessively.

# WHEEL BRIDGES

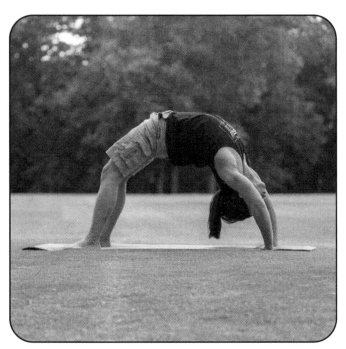

**ASCEND**

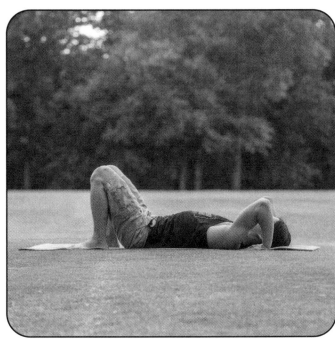

**DESCEND**

## TUTORIAL

1.  Lie on your back with your knees bent. Your heels should be a few inches away from your butt.

2.  Reach back until your palms touch the floor. Your hands should be next to your head with your fingers pointing towards your feet.

3.  Push through your palms and feet while arching your back until your arms and legs are as straight as you can make them. You should be in a Full Bridge position - supported only be your palms and feet!

4.  Pause for 10 Seconds. Use this time to stretch and move your body into place.

5.  Slowly reverse the movement.

6.  Pause for 10 Seconds.

7.  Repeat 3-6.

# STANDARDS

**LEVEL 1:** 2 Sets of 5
**LEVEL 2:** 2 Sets of 10
**LEVEL 3:** 2 Sets of 15

Do 2-3 sets of as many as you can.

Once you can meet or exceed Level 3 with **GOOD FORM,** you are ready to move on to a harder variation.

# BEHIND THE EXERCISE

You may have noticed that some Full Bridges don't quite look as aesthetically appealing as others.

This is because there's a significant difference between doing a Bridge and doing it well.

This step refers to the months-long process of improving our bridge. Gradually straightening the limbs is a good place to start. Focus on forming an "upside down letter U". Also learn to breathe normally throughout the exercise.

This is named after the Wheel Pose in yoga.

# FORM CUES

Video yourself doing these exercises and watch back in between sets. This can help all exercises!

Try to straighten your arms.

Try to straighten your legs.

Try to retract your scapula and bring your shoulders back.

Try to breathe normally.

Try to keep your bridge "even." Don't lean too far towards your feet or your palms. Try to keep it balanced. If your wrists hurt, you may need to move towards your palms a bit.

Try to arch your back evenly. Don't hinge at one point while keeping the rest straight. Imagine your back being as curved as the letter U upside down.

# PROGRESSION & REGRESSION

**To make this exercise harder:** Doing this exercise with perfect form is will make this exercise harder! Aim for straighter legs and arms. Breathe normally. Maintain a smooth curve in the back. Be an upside down U rather than an upside down V.

**To make this exercise easier:** Moving your hands and feet slightly further apart will make this exercise easier. You may need to lean towards your hands more so that your wrists don't have to bend excessively.

# TAP BRIDGES

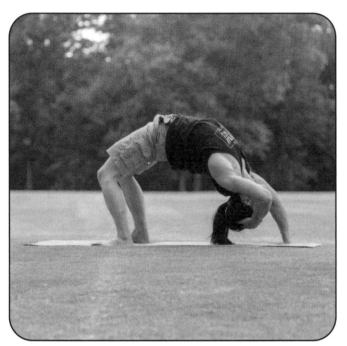

**ASCEND**

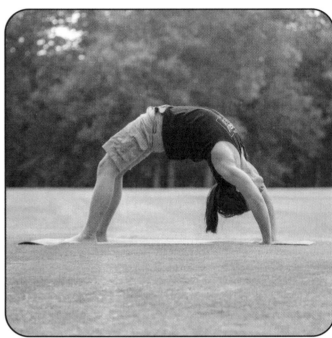

**DESCEND**

## TUTORIAL

1. Lie on your back with your knees bent. Your heels should be a few inches away from your butt.

2. Lean back and push yourself into a Wheel Bridge or Full Bridge.

3. Steadily shift weight onto one arm until you are able to lift the other arm entirely.

4. Tap your head or opposing shoulder briefly before returning your hand to the ground.

5. Repeat this motion for the other side.

6. Repeat 3-5.

## STANDARDS
(Per Side, Alternating)

**LEVEL 1:** 2 Sets of 5 Taps
**LEVEL 2:** 2 Sets of 20 Taps
**LEVEL 3:** 2 Sets of 30 Taps

Do 2-3 sets of as many as you can.

Once you can meet or exceed Level 3 with **GOOD FORM,** you are ready to move on to a harder variation.

# BEHIND THE EXERCISE

Theoretically, one could only use Wheel Bridges to improve their mobility until they are able to do Stand-to-Stand bridges.

However, it may be helpful to learn to assist oneself into the position with a wall.

This step gently introduces one-arm bridging that will be helpful for the next step. You may have trouble balancing at first. Don't fall on your head!

This exercise serves a quick "in-between" exercise to help us experiment with supporting our upper body with a single arm.

Provided you've spent solid time on the previous progressions, you may not need to spend much time on this exercise.

Follow this exercise with a few sets of Wheel Bridges to continue building your mobility.

# FORM CUES

Video yourself during this exercise and watch back in between sets. This can help all exercises!

Try to establish full balance with each "tap." If you feel like you have to rush to quickly touch your head and the ground again to avoid falling, spend extra time just learning to balance on your arms.

# PROGRESSION & REGRESSION

**To make this exercise harder:** Doing this exercise slower will make it more difficult. You can experiment with tapping your waist, your hips, etc. It doesn't really matter as long as you build the ability to balance on either arm.

**To make this exercise easier:** Quickly tapping yourself before returning to the floor will make this exercise easier. Make sure to practice this exercise until you're able to support yourself on either arm for at least a few seconds at any given time. This must feel stable for you to move to the next step.

# WALL WALKING BRIDGES

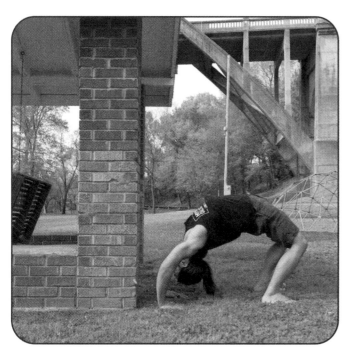

**ASCEND**

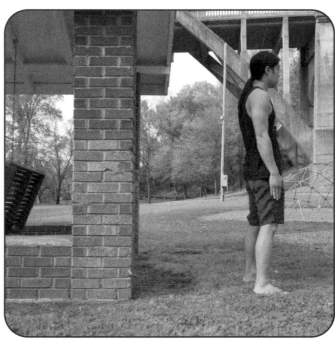

**DESCEND**

## TUTORIAL

1. Stand arm's length away from a stable wall. Your feet should be shoulder width apart.

2. Lean back steadily, start from your hips and "feeling" each vertebra move at a time, and place one palm on the wall behind you.

3. Do the same with your other palm, placing it slightly below the palm already on the wall.

4. Repeat this with each arm, "walking" yourself down the wall until your palms are on the ground in a Wheel Bridge or Full Bridge.

5. Take a deep breath to regain your bearings.

6. Lift one palm off the ground and place it securely against the wall.

7. Repeat the same with your other palm, placing it slightly above the palm already on the wall.

8. Repeat this with each arm until you are able to stand back up as you were in step 1.

9. Repeat 2-8.

# STANDARDS

**LEVEL 1:** 1 Sets of 3
**LEVEL 2:** 1 Sets of 6
**LEVEL 3:** 2 Sets of 10

Do 2-3 sets of as many as you can.

Once you can meet or exceed Level 3 with **GOOD FORM,** you are ready to move on to a harder variation.

# BEHIND THE EXERCISE

This exercise is basically assisting ourselves through the next goal in our Bridging journey: leaning back from a standing position to a Wheel Bridge position.

Using a wall to assist us from a standing position to a bridge position makes the transition easier.

Follow this exercise with a few sets of Wheel Bridges to continue building your mobility and range of motion.

IMPORTANT NOTE: Only attempt this step if you're able to meet the Level 3 standards all previous Bridge progressions - especially the Full Bridges and Wheel Bridges.

I know some people just browse the progressions to see which ones they can do, but an unprepared individual can seriously injure themselves on this exercise. Safety first!

# FORM CUES

Make sure your hands on the wall AND your feet on the ground are very secure. Don't wear only socks while doing this exercise. If you feel yourself "sliding" while leaning back, either go barefoot or find a wall, floor, and pair of shoes that allow you to be stable.

Try to establish full balance with each step. Do not rush to quickly go down the wall. This will only lead to injury.

Stand approximately arm's length away from the wall. Adjust as necessary.

Leaning back and placing the first hand may lead to dizziness even more than the previous exercises. Breathe normally. If dizziness occurs, stop and take a break.

# PROGRESSION & REGRESSION

**To make this exercise harder:** Using less assistance from your arms will make this exercise harder. You will know you're ready to move on when you barely need to touch the wall to lean back onto the floor.

**To make this exercise easier:** Using more assistance from your arms will make this exercise easier. If you have trouble descending all the way to the ground, stopping a few inches short might make the exercise easier.

# STAND TO STAND BRIDGES

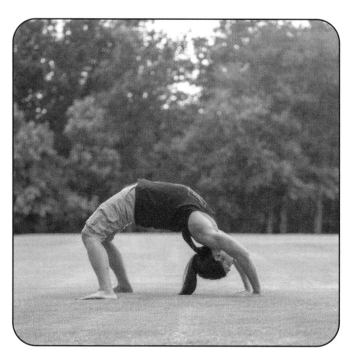

**ASCEND**

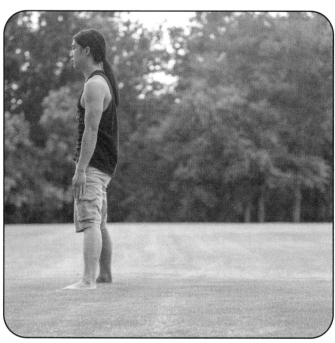

**DESCEND**

## TUTORIAL

1. Stand upright in a safe and secure location. Your feet should be shoulder width apart. Your hands should be on your hips.

2. Lean back steadily by pushing your hips forward and "feeling" each vertebra move at a time.

3. Keep leaning back until you are able to gently place one palm on the ground. You shouldn't need to fall on the palm.

4. After you are set, place your other palm on the ground. You should be in a Wheel Bridge or Full Bridge position.

5. Take a deep breath to regain your bearings.

6. Slowly reverse the movement by pushing through one palm and lifting the other until you are able to stand back up.

7. Place your hands back on your hips while you stand upright. Take a moment to gather your bearings.

8. Repeat 2-7.

# STANDARDS

**LEVEL 1:** 1 Set of 1
**LEVEL 2:** 1 Sets of 3
**LEVEL 3:** 2 Sets of 5

Do 2-3 sets of as many as you can.

Once you can meet or exceed Level 3 with **GOOD FORM,** you are ready to move on to a harder variation.

# BEHIND THE EXERCISE

Leaning back into a perfect Bridge is an incredible mobility feat.

While some are able to do this with "okay" form, strive to do this with excellent form!

Congratulations if you manage to make it here. Building up to this exercise progressively will keep your back healthy and strong for years to come. Do not attempt unless you've built up with previous exercises!

IMPORTANT NOTE: Only attempt this step if you're able to meet the Level 3 standards all previous Bridge progressions - especially the Full Bridges and Wheel Bridges.

I know some people just browse the progressions to see which ones they can do, but an unprepared individual can seriously injure themselves on this exercise. Safety first!

# FORM CUES

Make sure you are in a secure, safe area. No running kids, pets, or general hectic activity. You want to be able to focus for your own safety and balance.

This exercise is easier if you bend your knees or spread your feet far apart. Aim to do this exercise with your feet shoulder width apart and toes pointing forward or slightly out.

Leaning back and placing the first hand may lead to dizziness even more than the previous exercises. Breathe normally. If dizziness occurs, stop and take a break.

# PROGRESSION & REGRESSION

**To make this exercise harder:** Using a narrower stance as well as placing and pressing both palms at once will make this exercise harder. Some individuals may be able to do this exercise with straight legs!

**To make this exercise easier:** Leaning back on to a platform will make this exercise easier. You can lean onto a low bed or a couch. Just make sure it is safe and secure. A "springy" surface may cause some wrist pain as your wrists have to flex more. Additionally, using a wider stance will make this exercise easier.

# CLOSING THOUGHTS

Congratulations on working your way through the Bridge series! While the exercise is unconventional, it can help reverse some of the effects of sedentary behavior in modern life! Most of us spend so much time bending *forward*. Who would have thought we could balance this out by bending *back*?

If you build up gradually, you'll start to notice the many benefits of bridging. Unlike some of the other movements in this book, the bridging movement isn't really done much outside of exercise. However, you may notice better posture, more mobility, and even better energy!

It's not uncommon to want to explore beyond bridges. Here are some variations below. You way want to look them up online to get a better visual idea of how they're performed:

**Camel Poses -** For those who have trouble getting into a Full Bridge, this variation can offer very similar benefits! While on your knees, lean back slowly until your hands can rest gently on your heels or feet. This can be done for repetitions or as a hold!

**Bridge Holds -** Like almost any exercise, the Bridge can be done as an isometric exercise. For progression purposes, we measure repetitions for Full Bridges. However, they can also be done as holds! This is great for ironing out your technique because you get lots of time in the top position.

**Wall Slides / Wall Angels -** While not directly associated with Bridges, these exercises can be excellent for scapular mobility and posture.

Stand with your back to the wall. Try to keep your body as close to the wall as possible. Lift your arms up so that they are parallel to the ground, with your elbows bent and the back of your hands to the wall.

Slowly slide your arms up as high as you can, tightening your abs to prevent your lower back from arching, then slowly lower your arms back down to the starting position. Squeeze your arms back like you're trying to touch your shoulder blades. Repeat for repetitions. Try to keep your body as close to the wall as possible.

Warm up beforehand and don't stretch into areas of pain!

---

Don't rush through the steps. Many people will spend years just building up to Wheel Bridges. That variation will probably give the most benefit to most people. Especially ambitious individuals can (gradually and safely) work towards a Stand to Stand Bridge! This is an extra challenge of mobility and strength.

### Where do I start?

Start with a variation that you can do competently with good form for at least a few repetitions. When in doubt, start with Glute Bridges!

### I feel like I can't arch my back the way I need to for these exercises. How do I fix this?

You might need to work on mobility in your thoracic spine, or upper back. The Twists help improve the mobility of your spine, so be sure to incorporate these into your routine if you haven't already. Mobility can take time to train, so be patient and consistent.

There are also a number of gentle yoga poses that can help improve your mobility. Try warming up with cat-cow, downward dog, or cobra pose.

### I have met the standard for one variation, but the next exercise feels too hard. What should I do?

Each exercise has a Progression and a Regression. You can use these to your advantage!

For example, let's say you are stuck somewhere between two exercises. If your Wall Bridges are too easy, the Progression will challenge your body in preparation for the next exercise (stand farther away).

Alternatively, if the Incline Bridges are too challenging, the Regression will allow you to build into them more slowly (use a higher platform).

You can think of these as transition exercises!

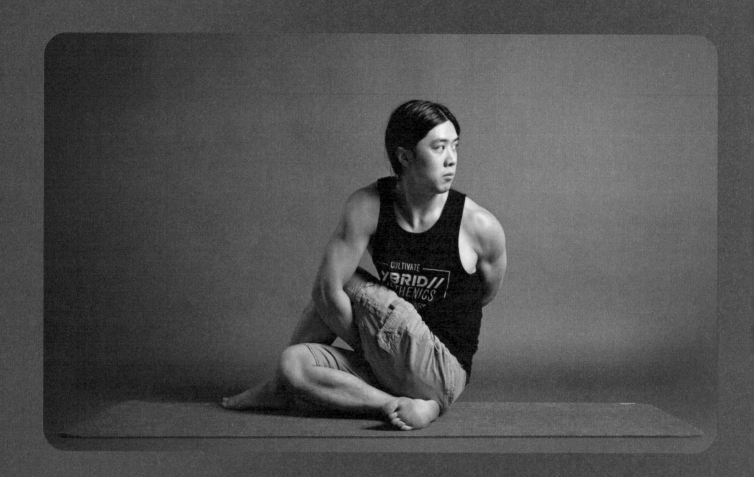

# TWISTS

The Twist is a bit of a different movement than the previous exercises we've covered. It's the only rotational movement listed here, and it's intended to improve mobility rather than strength.

Due to the linear nature of our daily movements, we tend to neglect rotational exercises. Mobility of the thoracic spine is quite functional. It helps us check out blind spots while merging on the freeway. It allows us to more evenly distribute the weight of

carrying our big brains around all day. Having a mobile spine improves the quality of your daily life!

Every Twist variation is a complex movement that works many muscles. These exercises stretch and contract the sides of our body — sometimes called the lateral chain. While these are static holds and not movements, you might notice you can really feel the stretching muscles as you breathe!

# GENERAL TWIST CUES

Progression is key for these exercises. See the "Progression & Regression" section for each exercise to find easier variations. It's normal to have multiple "mini progressions" before you are able to do the Full Twist.

It may help to bring some gentle full body exercises like jumping jacks or a jogging in place before doing these exercises. This will mobilize your musculature and make your stretch more effective.

Turn toward your RAISED BENT leg. This is helpful to align the movement. For some reason, it's easy to get confused on this. Many people initially turned toward their straight leg – myself possibly included.

Mind-muscle connection really matters here. Feel one side of your body stretch as the other side contracts. Small adjustments can help you feel the movement a lot better over the time you practice. This is one of the reasons longer holds are preferred.

Once you are in position, slightly look down as if you are trying to touch your chin to the shoulder toward which you are turning. This will help engage and stretch the muscles in the back of your neck.

You might feel some muscles near your hip cramp. If this happens, ease off the stretch and massage them a bit. Walk around. Then go back to your Twists.

Go slowly and steadily. Under NO circumstances should you use SPEED to twist into the movement or extend your range of motion. This would be a recipe for disaster. If you use control, your own body will regulate the safety of the movement.

# TWIST PROGRESSIONS

There may be only three variations to master, but progressing from Straight Leg Twists all the way to Full Twists will take patience and consistency. Remember to be intentional with your twists - it should feel like work, not like a relaxing stretch. Mastery of each variation will be hard won and worth it!

1. Straight Leg Twists
2. Bent Leg Twists
3. Full Twists

# STRAIGHT LEG TWISTS

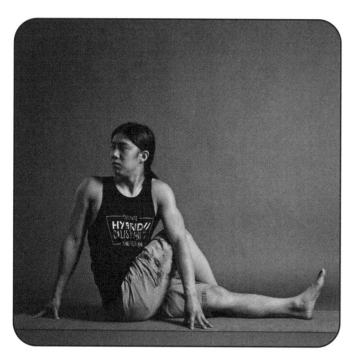

**FRONT**

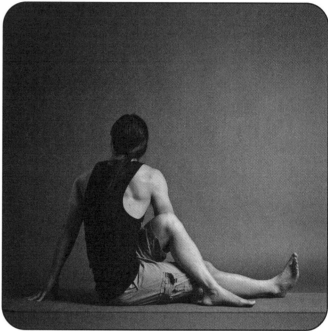

**BACK**

## TUTORIAL

1. Sit on the floor with your legs straight in front of you.

2. Place your right foot beside your left knee and cross it over so the foot is on the other side of the knee to your left.

3. Turn towards your bent leg and place your left hand on your right side.. Place your right hand behind you.

4. Continue turning to your right as hard as you safely can.

5. Breathe normally and hold for time.

6. Return to your starting position and do the exact same for the left side.

7. After doing both sides, rest 30 seconds before repeating again. See Standards.

## STANDARDS
(Both Sides)

**LEVEL 1:** 3 Holds of 15 Seconds
**LEVEL 2:** 3 Holds of 30 Seconds
**LEVEL 3:** 3 Holds of 60 Seconds

Do 2-3 sets of as many as you can.

Once you can meet or exceed Level 3 with **GOOD FORM,** you are ready to move on to a harder variation.

# BEHIND THE EXERCISE

An introduction to twisting. Twist as hard as you safely can.

Think of this a mobility exercise - not necessarily a relaxation exercise.

# FORM CUES

Turn toward your BENT leg. This is helpful to align the movement. For some reason, it's easy to get confused on this. Many people initially turned toward their straight leg - myself possibly included.

# PROGRESSION & REGRESSION

**To make this exercise harder:** Slowly experiment with bending your straight leg will make this exercise harder (see Bent Knee Twists). Don't bend your leg halfway and attempt to make progress this way. This puts unnecessary sideways pressure on the knee. Bend your knee all the way and attempt twisting with proper posture.

**To make this exercise easier:** If you are unable to place your hand on the outside of your knee, simply turning without involving your arms will make this exercise easier. You will know you are making progress when you can place your elbow on the outside of your knee.

# BENT LEG TWISTS

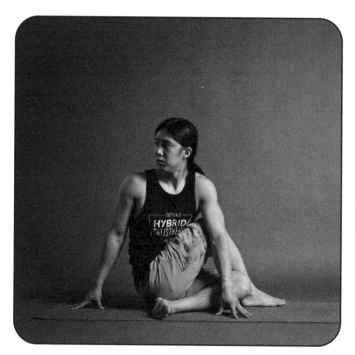

**FRONT**

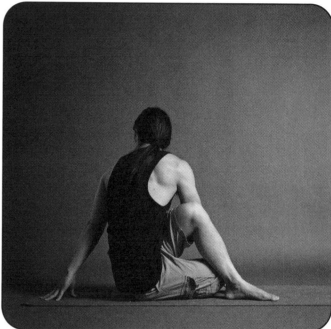

**BACK**

## TUTORIAL

1.  Sit on the floor with your legs straight in front of you.

2.  Place your right foot beside your left knee and cross it over so the foot is on the other side of the knee to your left.

3.  Bend your left knee and place your left heel on your right butt cheek.

4.  Turn towards your bent leg and place your left hand on your right side.. Place your right hand behind you.

5.  Continue turning to your right as hard as you safely can.

6.  Breathe normally and hold for time.

7.  Return to your starting position and do the exact same for the left side.

8.  After doing both sides, rest 30 seconds before repeating again. See Standards.

## STANDARDS
(Both Sides)

**LEVEL 1:** 3 Holds of 15 Seconds
**LEVEL 2:** 3 Holds of 30 Seconds
**LEVEL 3:** 3 Holds of 60 Seconds

Do 2-3 sets of as many as you can.

Once you can meet or exceed Level 3 with **GOOD FORM,** you are ready to move on to a harder variation.

# BEHIND THE EXERCISE

Touching the leg increases the mobility demands!

This also brings our hips into the stretch. You may feel some tight muscles in your glutes and on the side of your hips finally start to loosen up.

# FORM CUES

You might feel some muscles near your hip cramp. If this happens, ease off the stretch and massage them a bit. Walk around. Then go back to your Twists.

It may help you to jog in place a bit before this exercise. This may help loosen up some lower body muscles and improve this exercise's effectiveness.

# PROGRESSION & REGRESSION

**To make this exercise harder:** Twisting more will make this exercise harder. It may be helpful to view the next exercise - Full Twists - to see the goal and know where your body has to go. You can experiment with placing one hand underneath the raised leg. This will stretch your shoulder external rotators and prepare you for the next step!

**To make this exercise easier:** Twisting less will make this exercise easier.

# FULL TWISTS

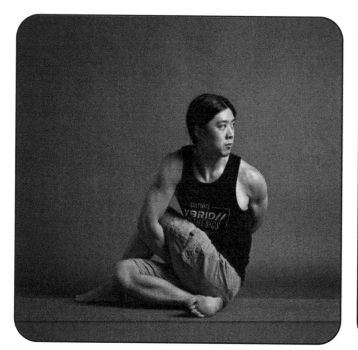

**FRONT**

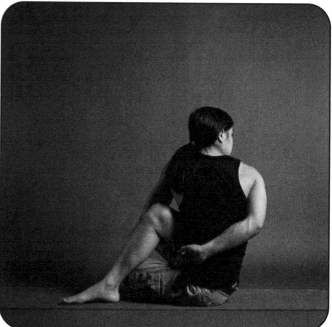

**BACK**

## TUTORIAL

1. Sit on the floor with your legs straight in front of you.
2. Place your right foot beside your left knee and cross it over so the foot is on the other side of the knee to your left.
3. Bend your left knee and place your left heel on your right butt cheek.
4. Turn slowly towards your bent leg.
5. Thread your left arm under your right knee from the outside.
6. Turn a bit more towards the right until you are able to grab your left hand with your right hand.
7. Hold your hands together while turning as hard as you safely can to the right side.
8. Breathe normally and hold for time.
9. Return to your starting position and do the exact same for the left side.
10. After doing both sides, rest 30 seconds before repeating again. See Standards.

## STANDARDS
(Both Sides)

**LEVEL 1:** 3 Holds of 15 Seconds
**LEVEL 2:** 3 Holds of 30 Seconds
**LEVEL 3:** 3 Holds of 60 Seconds

Do 2-3 sets of as many as you can.

Once you can meet or exceed Level 3 with **GOOD FORM,** you are ready to move on to a harder variation.

# BEHIND THE EXERCISE

Linking arms is an exceptional mobility standard! Congratulations!

Regular practice of this will bolster joint mobility and iron out muscular imbalance. Your back will be stronger and more mobile for years to come. Congratulations!

Full Twists have all the benefits of the previous progressions. "Threading" your arms together brings the stretch to our rotator cuff - often stiff and weak from misuse.

# FORM CUES

Progression is key to this exercise. See the "Progression & Regression" section on this page to find easier variations. It's normal to have multiple "mini progressions" before you are able to do the Full Twist.

It may help to bring some gentle full body exercises like jumping jacks before doing this exercise. This will mobilize your musculature and make your stretch more effective.

# PROGRESSION & REGRESSION

**To make this exercise harder:** Like with all Twists, twisting more will make this exercise more difficult. After a lot of practice, you may be able to hold wrists instead of hands. Take care to make sure every inch of your Twist is controlled. Remember this is simply a mobility exercise that also conditions the sides of our body. There's not much benefit to extreme levels of twisting.

**To make this exercise easier:** Joining your hands together is exceptionally difficult. It may help you to use a rope or hand towel. See the video above for reference.

# CLOSING THOUGHTS

Congratulations on working your way through the Twist series! If you can do Full Twists comfortably, you've built much more rotational mobility that the average person.

If you can't yet, that's okay too! I mean... did you just skip to the end of this section or near the end of the book out of curiosity?

(That's fine if you did. This book isn't meant to be read linearly. If it was, it'd take most people years to finish all the variations).

Jokes aside, you may have noticed that the Twist section is different from other sections of the book. For starters, there are only three progressions. Also, we're counting seconds instead of repetitions! What gives?? *cue dramatic music*

This is because the Twists are meant to be trained in a very self-regulated manner. Some readers may struggle with Straight Leg Twists. Perhaps they can only reach halfway towards what I demonstrate in the photos.

Good news — that's okay! These twists are rotational stretches. So as long as you're feeling the stretch, the exercise is working its intended function. You may want to warm up beforehand for optimal results. Avoid stretching into areas of pain! Especially for your neck. As usual, we want to start slow. We only have one spine, so we should take care of it.

There are different ways you can harness and enhance the rotational function you gather from Twists:

**Punching –** If you have access to a punching bag or a safe punching surface, this can be a great workout! If you've never punched anything before, you may want to look up a quick guide on technique so you don't injure yourself. Also, for the purposes of this book, only punch things you're legally allowed to punch.

**Kicking –** The same as above, but with your lower body!

**Throwing –** This is underrated! If you can find a safe area, tossing a ball at a tree or wall can help you feel how rotation enhances your throwing ability. For an added challenge, try throwing with your non-dominant arm.

---

These example movements are fun — but optional. If you were especially stiff beforehand, they help you feel the newfound freedom that additional mobility may give you. Explore this if you want!

## Where do I start?

Start with a variation that you can do competently with good form for at least a few repetitions. When in doubt, start with Straight Leg Twists!

## I can do the twist, but I have trouble keeping my hands on the ground. Is that okay?

For some of us, placing or keeping our hands on the ground is going to be extra challenging. Try your best to master the form, and be patient with it! Mobility takes time to build.

## I have met the standard for one variation, but the next exercise feels too hard. What should I do?

Each exercise has a Progression and a Regression. You can use these to your advantage!

For example, let's say you are stuck somewhere between the first two exercises. If your Straight Leg Twists are too easy, the Progression will challenge your body in preparation for the next exercise (trying it with a bent leg).

Alternatively, if the Bent Leg Twists are too challenging, the Regression will allow you to build into them more slowly (twisting less).

You can think of these as transition exercises!

## I have trouble with Straight Leg Twists. I can't twist as far as the photos show.

That's okay. The stretch will look slightly different for different people. For Twists, just rotate as far as you safely can to feel the stretch.

## I have trouble keeping time or counting the seconds.

You can use a clock, watch, or timer. Most smartphones have this capability. However, some people prefer to count their breaths instead of seconds. This is fine too. Take note of how often you take breaths and use this to calculate the seconds. It doesn't have to be exact.

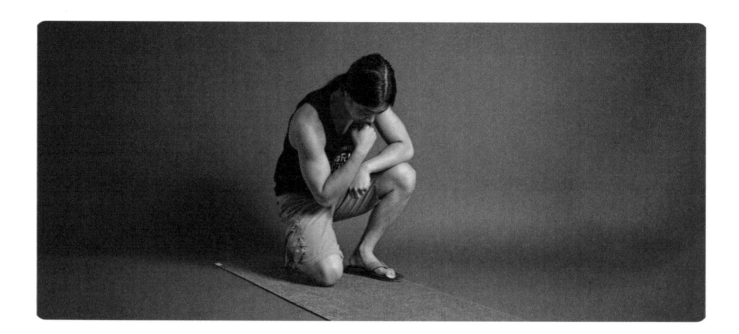

## HELP! I DON'T KNOW HOW TO GET STARTED!

That's okay. We've got you covered! If you're just starting out you should begin with the first of each exercise. Building a strong foundation is very important for everything that comes afterward!

Take a look at the Hybrid Routine 2.0, then take a look at your schedule. Where does your workout fit? Can you add it to your calendar, or maybe set an alarm? What barriers might get in your way, and how can you tackle them? Set yourself up for success by thinking ahead and making a plan of action!

### I don't have a place to attach gym rings or install a pullup bar. What are my options?

It's tough to replace the Full Pullup with a different bodyweight exercise. You can try using a sturdy table or a pair of sturdy chairs to do horizontal pullups, or inverted rows. Some use a sturdy stick between two couches. These exercises will target the muscle group in a similar manner. Just make sure your set up is safe!

However, it's well worth it to find something you can use for Full Pullups. Check out your local park and see if there are some monkey bars around!

## I am experiencing pain/discomfort in my _____ . How do I address this?

If an exercise or a movement is painful for you, stop the exercise or dial it back to a non-painful level. Whether it's brand new or has been happening for years, it's always a good idea to see a doctor.

## I have been working out for _____ days/weeks and I feel like I'm not making progress. What am I doing wrong?

You might not be doing anything wrong at all! Change takes time, and patience is a challenging exercise. If you are following the routine closely, you have double-checked your form, and you are getting the right nutrition, it may simply be a matter of time.

## I have met the standard for one variation, but the next exercise feels too hard. What should I do?

Each exercise has a Progression and a Regression. You can use these to your advantage!

For example, let's say you are stuck somewhere between two exercises. If your Wall Bridges are too easy, the Progression will challenge your body in preparation for the next exercise (stand farther away).

Alternatively, if the Incline Bridges are too challenging, the Regression will allow you to build into them more slowly (use a higher platform).

You can think of these as transition exercises!

## I'm having trouble keeping my heels on the ground during my squats. How can I fix this?

You might need to work on your ankle flexibility! You can do this by going back to the first variations and focusing solely on your range of motion. Try moving slowly and pausing at the bottom to train in proper heel placement.

You can also do calf stretches in between your sets to improve your flexibility.

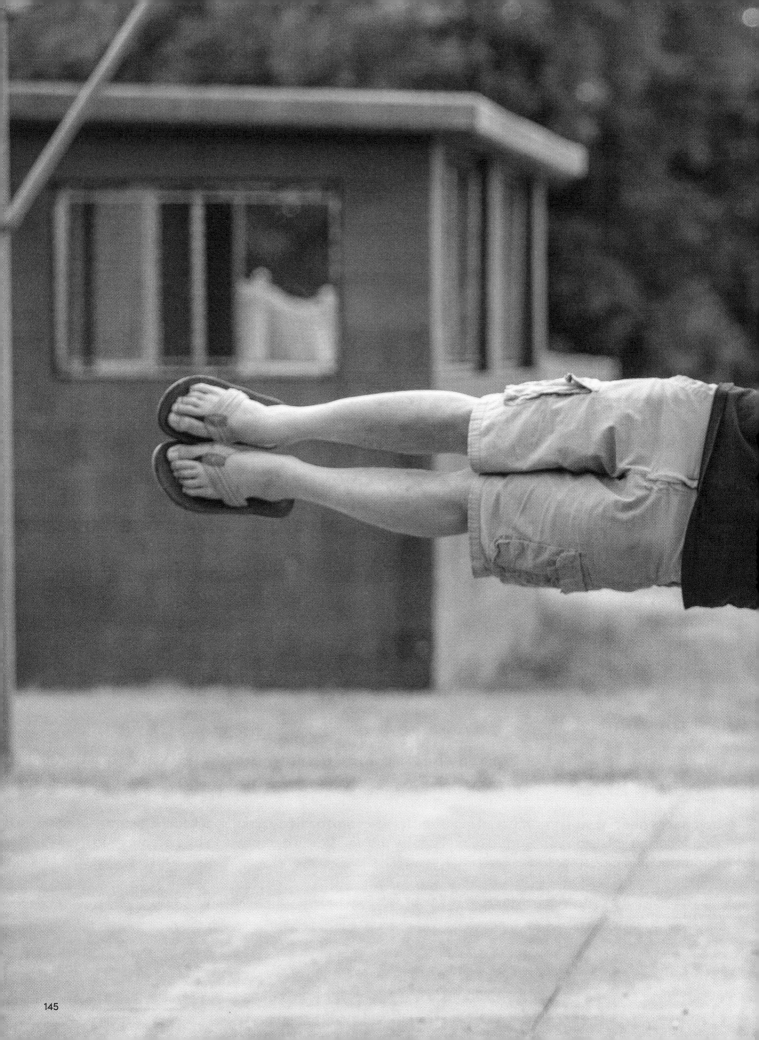

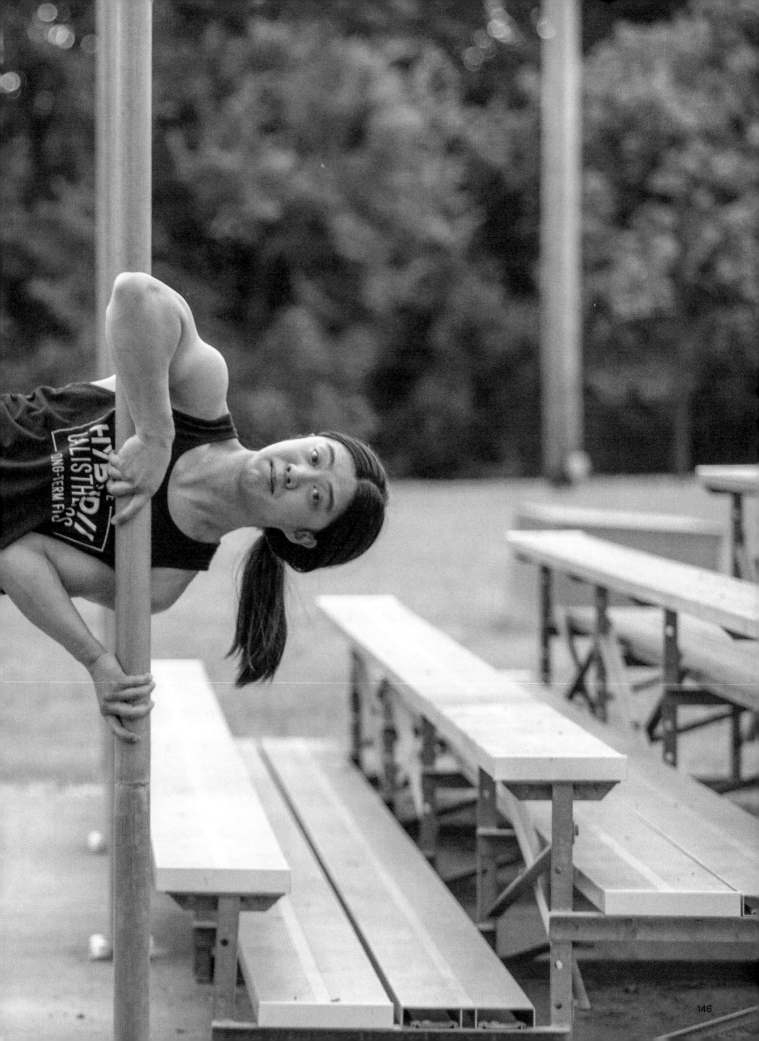

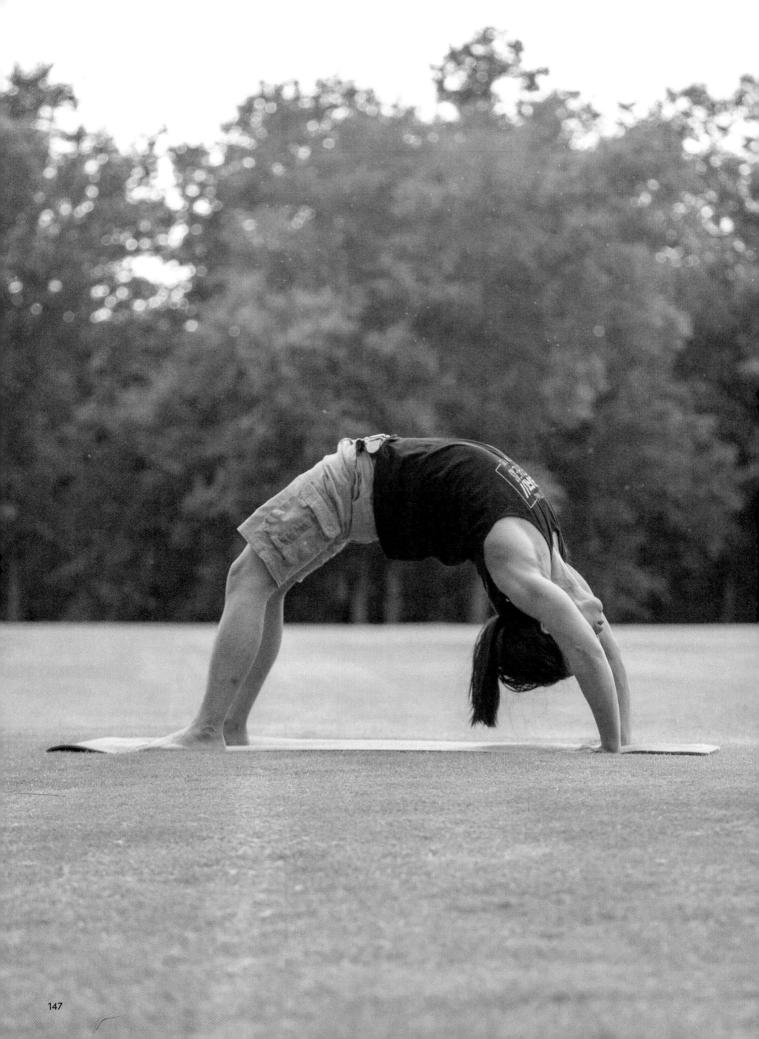

# CONCLUSION

## THAT'S IT FOR NOW!

Thank you for reading! If you read the entirety of this book, it represents a simple, scalable way for almost anybody in the world to get physically fit. After you understand the concepts, you can use them to make progress for the rest of your life! You can also teach them to others, if you choose.

Of course, finishing this book through reading is different from actually "finishing" the routine, right? It can take years to scale through all the exercises and do them competently! If you get bored with it, feel free to try other things. Add to your routine. Change it. Improve it. Stick it in a stew (maybe not that).

You can always come back and pick up where you left off! The floor and gravity aren't going anywhere. I hope, anyway.

That said, consistency is key to progress! Balance your curiosity with dedication for long-term results.

### Support

Progress is rarely a straight line. As you might have already discovered, fitness routines leave room for confusion. Maybe you have a question about joint angles. Or perhaps you don't "feel" like an exercise is working.

Thankfully, you're not alone in doing the Hybrid Routine! Thousands of people do it every week – just like you can! Check out our website, online communities, and support resources below!

**Website:** www.hybridcalisthenics.com
**Email:** support@hybridcalisthenics.com

—

Have a beautiful day, my friend!